Diagnostic Imaging in Clinical Medicine (ISSN 0254-881X), **Vol. 55, No. 1-2 (1986)**
Editor: Wm. Penn, Oud-Turnhout

Symposium on Magnetic Resonance, Utrecht, April 26, 1985

Magnetic Resonance

Indications for Imaging and Considerations on the Other Possibilities

Editor: Wm. Penn, Oud-Turnhout

Based on a symposium organized by the Netherlands' Society of Diagnostic Radiology, this special issue surveys recent developments in Magnetic Resonance Imaging (MRI). Due to the increasing importance of this complex modality in daily radiological practice, contributions emphasize not only the basic principles, but also the practical uses of MRI in the brain, spine, heart, genitourinary tract, and orbit and knee. The issue also contains several papers showing how the quality of magnetic resonance images can be improved by the use of optimal field strength, proton chemical shift imaging and the application of special MR contrast media. A further topic discussed is the use of nuclear magnetic resonance spectroscopy which, although it has not yet lived up to its promise as a clinical tool, is established as an important tool of biomedical research. Taken together, these papers provide clinical radiologists with interesting information on the indications of MRI and its absolute and relative advantages over other forms of diagnostic imaging.

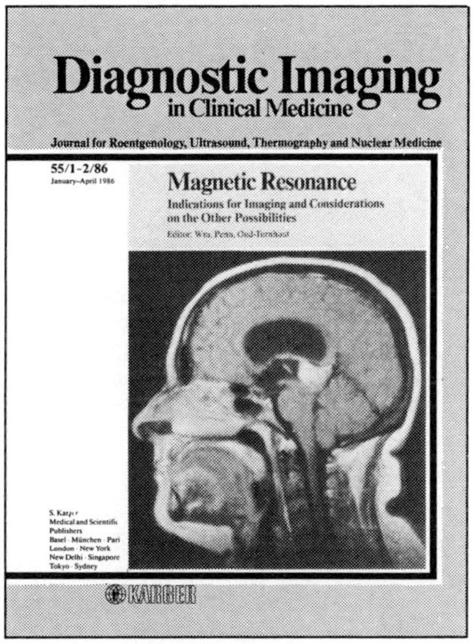

Field of Interest
Radiology

Contents

Diagnostic Imaging in Clinical Medicine, Vol. 55, No. 1-2 (1986)
Magnetic Resonance
Indications for Imaging and Considerations for the Other Possibilities
Symposium on Magnetic Resonance, Utrecht, April 26, 1985
Editor.: Wm. Penn, Oud-Turnhout
108 p., 77 fig., 3 color pl., 17 tab., soft cover, 1986
SFr. 88.- / DM 105.- / US $ 49.00
ISBN 3-8055-4259-3

KARGER

KI 85281

Contributions to Nephrology (ISSN 0302–5144), **Vol. 49**
Series Editors: G.M. Berlyne, Brooklyn, N.Y.; S. Giovannetti, Pisa

Volume Editors:
A. Amerio; P. Coratelli, Bari;
V.M. Campese; S.G. Massry,
Los Angeles, Calif.

Metabolic and Endocrine Disturbances in Renal Diseases

This volume will provide nephrologists, endocrinologists and internists with an update review of selected topics in basic and clinical nephrology.

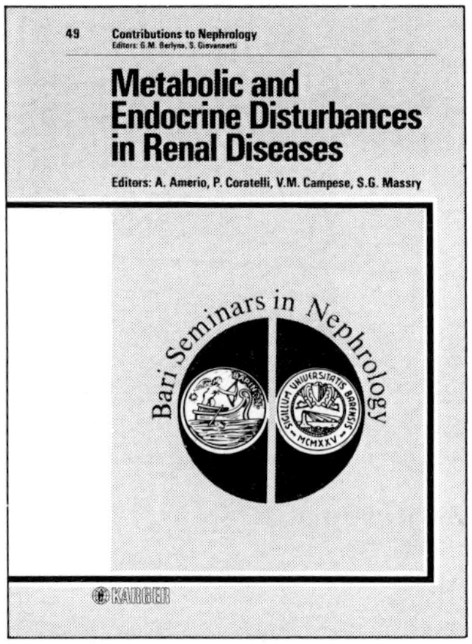

The most recent concerns on the metabolic and endocrine disturbances frequently observed in renal patients are reviewed in this work. The 26 papers, based on presentations from a congress, are grouped under three major headings: Metabolism and Endocrine Disturbances; Nephrolithiasis; Hormones, Kidneys and Hypertension.
In the first section, evidence is presented supporting the concept of PTH as a major uremic toxin which exhibits a causative effect on hormonal imbalances and disturbances in lipid metabolism. Dietary management of the uremic patient is carefully assessed in two studies investigating the effects of a protein restricted diet on both testicular endocrine function and on the progression rate of chronic renal failure. Management of iron overload in chronic hemodialysis is difficult, however desferrioxamine is shown to be the most effective chelator available for treatment. The causes and treatment of nephrolithiasis are reviewed in the second section. Studies suggest animal protein consumption is a major determinant in the risk for nephrolithiasis. The biologic activities of thiazide, and the clinical effects of its long-term administration to patients with recurrent calcium nephrolithiasis, are summarized. Incidence and type of metabolic disturbances associated with an increased risk of calculi formation are reviewed. The third group of chapters assesses the role of the adrenergic system, prostaglandins, the kidneys, and minerals on arterial hypertension.

Contents

Metabolic and Endocrine Disturbances
with contributions by S.G. Massry; T. Drüeke and B. Lacour; P. Coratelli et al.; K. Olgaard et al.; M. Olmer et al.; J. Kovarik et al.; N.G. DeSanto et al.; G. Barsotti et al.; V. Bonomini et al.; N. Gretz and M. Strauch; G. Carmelo et al.

Nephrolithiasis
with contributions by W. Tschöpe and E. Ritz; A. Ulmann and J. Clavel; G. Maschio et al.; B. Baggio et al.; A. Jeantet et al.

Hormones, Kidneys and Hypertension
with contributions by V.M. Campese and S.G. Massry; A. Zuccalà et al.; J. Hagege et al.; V.M. Campese; G.G. Neri Serneri et al.; G. Bianchi et al.; G. Masotti et al.; D.C. Schohn et al.; J. Kindler et al.; A. Heidland et al.

Contributions to Nephrology, Vol. 49
Metabolic and Endocrine Disturbances in Renal Diseases
Bari Seminars in Nephrology on Metabolic and Endocrine Disturbances in Renal Diseases, Bari, March 1984
Volume Editors: A. Amerio; P. Coratelli, Bari; V.M. Campese; S.G. Massry, Los Angeles, Calif.
VIII + 224 p., 47 fig., 41 tab., hard cover, 1985
SFr. 93.– / DM 111.– / US $ 39.75
DM / US $ prices subject to change
ISBN 3-8055-4143-0

KARGER

KI 85243

European Urology

Official Organ of the European Association of Urology

KARGER

Eur. Urol.
Printed in Switzerland

S. Karger AG,
Postfach, CH–4009 Basel (Schweiz)

Erscheint zweimonatlich;
pro Jahr 1 Band zu 6 Heften

Submission: Only original papers written in English are considered and should be sent to:

Prof. C.C. Schulman
Department of Urology
Hôpital Erasme
Cliniques Universitaires de Bruxelles
Route de Lennik 808
B-1070 Brussels (Belgium)

Manuscripts should be submitted in *triplicate* (with three sets of illustrations of which one is an original), typewritten double-spaced on one side of the paper, with a wide margin.

Conditions: All manuscripts are subject to editorial review. Manuscripts are received with the explicit understanding that they are not under simultaneous consideration by any other publication. Submission of an article for publication implies the transfer of the copyright from the author to the publisher upon acceptance. Accepted papers become the permanent property of 'European Urology' and may not be reproduced by any means, in whole or in part, without the written consent of the publisher. It is the author's responsibility to obtain permission to reproduce illustrations, tables, etc. from other publications.

Arrangement:

Title page: The first page of each paper should indicate the title (main title underlined), the authors' names, and the institute where the work was conducted. A short title for use as running head is also required.

Key words: For indexing purposes, a list of 3-10 key words in English is essential.

Abstract: Each paper needs an abstract of up to 10 lines.

Small type: Paragraphs which can or must be set in smaller type (case histories, test methods, etc.) should be indicated with a 'p' (petit) in the margin on the left-hand side.

Footnotes: Avoid footnotes. When essential, they are numbered consecutively and typed at the foot of the appropriate page.

Tables and illustrations: Tables (numbered in Roman numerals) and illustrations (numbered in Arabic numerals) should be prepared on separate sheets. Tables require a heading, and figures a legend, also prepared on a separate sheet. For the reproduction of illustrations, only good drawings and original photographs can be accepted; negatives or photocopies cannot be used. When possible, group several illustrations on one block for reproduction (max. size 176 × 224 mm) or provide crop marks. On the back of each illustration, indicate its number, the author's name, and 'top'. Color illustrations are reproduced at the author's expense.

References: The list of references should include only those publications which are cited in the text. References may be arranged alphabetically (citation by name and year) or numbered consecutively (citation by number).

a) Papers published in periodicals: 1. All authors' surnames ('et al.' is not sufficient) with initials of first names; 2. Full title of paper; 3. Journal abbreviation; 4. Volume (in Arabic numerals, underlined and followed by a colon); 5. First and last page; 6. Year of publication in brackets. Example: McIntosh, J.; Hansen, P.; Ziegler, J.; Penny, R.: Defective immune and phagocytic functions in uraemia and renal transplantation. Int. Archs Allergy appl. Immun. 51: 529-540 (1976).

b) Books: 1. Authors' surnames with initials of first names; 2. Full title; 3. In brackets, name and domicile of publisher and year of publication. Example: Pollack, R.S.: Tumor surgery of the head and neck (Karger, Basel 1975).

Full address: The exact postal address complete with postal code of the senior author must be given. If correspondence is handled by someone else, indicate this accordingly.

Further details: Authors may consult our leaflet 'Rules for the Preparation of Manuscripts', available on request from the Publisher, S. Karger AG, P.O. Box, CH-4009 Basel (Switzerland).

Page charges: There is no page charge for papers of 4 or fewer printed pages (including tables, illustrations and references). Each additional complete or partial page is charged to the author at SFr. 195.- / US$100.00. The allotted size of a paper is equal to approx. 15 manuscript pages (including tables, illustrations and references).

Galley proofs: Unless indicated otherwise, galley proofs are sent to the first-named author and should be returned with the least possible delay. Alterations made in galley proofs, other than the correction of printer's errors, are charged to the author. No page proofs are supplied.

Reprints: Order forms and a price list are sent with the galley proofs. Orders submitted after the issue is printed are subject to considerably higher prices. Allow five weeks from date of publication for normal delivery of reprints (airmail on request and at charge).

General Information

Publication data: 'European Urology' is published 6 times annually. Volume 12 with 6 issues appears in 1986.

Subscription rates: Subscriptions run for a full calendar year. Prices are given per volume, surface postage included.

Personal subscription: SFr. 277.20, US$150.50. (Must be in the name of, billed to, and paid by an individual. Order must be marked 'personal subscription'.)

Institutional subscription: SFr. 396.-, US$215.00. (Regular rate.)

Members of the European Association of Urology: SFr. 217.80, US$118.25.

Airmail postage: SFr. 30.-, US$ 15.00. (Extra per volume.)

Microform subscription: SFr. 198.-, US$ 94.50. (Available exclusively to subscribers of the paper edition.)

Single issues and back volumes: Information on availability and prices can be obtained through the Publisher.

Subscription orders: Orders can be placed at agencies, bookstores, directly with the Publisher S. Karger AG, P.O. Box, CH-4009 Basel (Switzerland) or with any of the following distributors:

Deutschland, West-Berlin, Ost-Europa, Naher Osten: S. Karger GmbH, Postfach 1724, D-8034 Germering/München

France: Librairie Luginbühl, 36, bd de Latour-Maubourg, F-75007 Paris

Great Britain: John Wiley and Sons, Ltd., Baffins Lane, Chichester, Sussex, PO19 1UD

USA: S. Karger Publishers, Inc., 79 Fifth Avenue, New York, NY 10003

India, Bangladesh, Sri Lanka: S. Karger India Subscription Agency, B-5/132 Safdarjung Enclave, New Delhi-110029

Japan, South Korea: Katakura Libri, Inc., 36-9 Hongo 3-chome, Bunkyo-ku, Tokyo 113

Change of address: Both old and new address should be stated and sent to the subscription source.

Bibliographic indices: This journal is regularly listed in bibliographic services, including *Current Contents®*.

Book Reviews: Books are accepted for review by special agreement.

Advertising: Correspondence and rate requests should be addressed to the Publisher.

KARGER

Laser in Urology

Proceedings of the

International Symposium Laser in Urology

Lübeck, November 9, 1985

Guest Editor:
A. Hofstetter, Lübeck

48 figures and 11 tables, 1986

KARGER

S. Karger · Medical and Scientific Publishers · Basel · München · Paris · London · New York · New Delhi · Singapore · Tokyo · Sydney

Drug Dosage

The authors and the publisher have exerted every effort to ensure that drug selection and dosage set forth in this text are in accord with current recommendations and practice at the time of publication. However, in view of ongoing research, changes in government regulations, and the constant flow of information relating to drug therapy and drug reactions, the reader is urged to check the package insert for each drug for any change in indications and dosage and for added warnings and precautions. This is particularly important when the recommended agent is a new and/or infrequently employed drug.

Printed in Switzerland by Graphische Anstalt Schüler AG, Biel
ISBN 3-8055-4362-X

Contents

Introduction

This symposium presented a good overview of the present-day possibilities of the neodymium-YAG laser used in urology.

Frank (Munich) first presented an introduction to the physics and biophysics of the major lasers at present employed in the field of medicine. It was seen that, on the basis of the ability of the neodymium-YAG laser to produce deep 'voluminous' necroses and the possibility of being able to use it under water, this laser is ideal for endoscopic tumor destruction.

The presentation of the most important laser endoscopes was followed by a discussion of safety aspects. Here, the most important point was that, in contrast to open laser applications, endoscopic work employing rigid instruments does not require special protective glasses for the eyes.

Since the best-studied application of the laser is the treatment of tumors of the bladder, this latter was at the center of interest. The histopathological changes brought about by the neodymium-YAG laser irradiation of bladder and liver tissue were demonstrated by Keiditsch (Munich), it being particularly worth emphasizing that, with the neodymium-YAG laser, accurately defined volume necroses can be produced in the tissue. Surprisingly, the experimental results reported by Pensel (Lübeck), who used the neodymium-YAG laser to produce extensive necroses in the bladders of rabbits, showed that the necrotic tissue was replaced not merely by connective tissue, but also by muscle tissue. This might, perhaps, explain why, after extensive neodymium-YAG laser irradiation of the human bladder, no atrophy of the bladder has so far been observed.

Hofstetter (Lübeck) reported on a prospective, randomized, and controlled study initiated in 1981 comparing the effect of the neodymium-YAG laser and transurethral tumor resection. Here, it was clearly shown that the neodymium-YAG laser reduces the incidence of recurrent disease and prolongs the recurrence-free interval. This was demonstrated both for primary and recurrent tumors. The same results were found, independently, by Maier's working group (Vienna), so that the application of the neodymium-YAG laser in tumors of the bladder may be considered a real advance.

But it is not merely tumors of the bladder that respond well to treatment with the neodymium-YAG laser – also tumors of the renal parenchyma, the pelvicalyceal system, the ureter and the urethra, and also of the external genitals. Thus, Hutschenreiter (Duisburg-Oberhausen) reported on his experience with the neodymium-YAG laser in the treatment of carcinomas of the renal pelvis. Because of the small number of cases involved and his, as yet, relatively limited experience, he described the technique as palliative. In contrast, Böwering and Schilling (Munich) reported on excellent results achieved with the neodymium-YAG laser in the treatment of carcinomas of the ureter and renal pelvis, with reference to our case material at the hospital in the Thalkirchener Strasse, Munich, which includes follow-up periods of more than 4 years.

Rothenberger (Landshut) submitted patients we had treated – also a number of years ago in Munich – for carcinomas of the penis to follow-up examinations and was able to establish that, over a 5-year observation period, we had lost only 1 of a total of 18 patients to this disease. This patient had refused to undergo regional lymph node dissection. This would mean that, in the case of carcinoma of the penis, we have achieved a 5-year survival rate of more than 90% – using only local laser therapy.

With respect to new fields of application of the neodymium-YAG laser, Beisland and Sander (Oslo) reported on the possible use of the laser to treat carcinoma of the prostate. After 1 year, the results were excellent – which, however, does not mean that we have to await longer observation periods before we are able to take up a definitive position or to recommend this technique.

Tansey and Shanberg (Los Angeles) reported on the possibilities of using the laser for prostatotomy and for treating interstitial cystitis.

Schmiedt and Jocham (Munich) presented their concept of integral photoradiotherapy in multifocal bladder carcinoma. However, the number of clinical cases was very small, and the observation period short, so that it is, at present, not possible to make a final evaluation, in particular in comparison with the neodymium-YAG laser.

Benson (Rochester) who has been working on this problem for years, expressed the opinion that this technique has only a very limited indication – for superficial carcinomas of the bladder.

Finally, Frank (Munich) reported on our initial experience with laser-induced intracorporeal shock wave lithotripsy, which possibly represents a new approach to the treatment of stones, which certainly should not be considered a rival to extracorporeal shock wave lithotripsy, but, rather, a useful supplement, in particular in the case of stones in the ureter.

This symposium has shown that the continuous-wave neodymium-YAG laser has proven extremely useful for endoscopic and open destruction of tumors, that as a Q-switched laser it may possibly soon be available for the treatment of ureteral, bladder and perhaps also renal stones and gallstones, and that there might also be other applications for it, such as, for example, angioplasty. But despite the quite astonishing results that have so far been achieved with the neodymium-YAG laser, it should not be forgotten that the laser can be considered a suitable surgical instrument only when its application is really indicated.

A. Hofstetter, Lübeck

Eur. Urol. *12:* suppl. 1, pp. 3–11 (1986)

0302–2838/86/0127–0003$2.75/0

Biophysical Fundamentals, Technical Prerequisites, and Safety Aspects for the Application of the Neodymium-YAG Laser in Urology

F. Frank

MBB-Medizintechnik GmbH, Applikationsforschung, München, BRD

Key Words. Nd:YAG laser · Tissue denaturation · Coagulation · Light guides · Laser cystoscope · Laser safety

Abstract. The relationship between the physical parameters of the biological objects and the parameters of the laser radiation is important when considering the interaction between laser radiation and biological molecules. A consideration of the dependence of absorption and scattering in the tissue on wavelength alone permits a simple explanation of the various thermal effects of the various laser systems used in surgery. The thermal properties of tissue may be assumed to be the same as those of water. As an example of a medical neodymium-YAG laser instrument the mediLas system is presented with different application instruments that are necessary for an efficient use of the laser. The prerequisite for the use of high-power laser in surgery is complete safety not only for the patient when determining the right irradiation dose, but also for the doctor and his staff.

Introduction

The principle of Light Amplification by Stimulated Emission of Radiation, i.e., the LASER, has now been known since 1960. The rapid development of a variety of different laser systems has led to a wide range of uses.

Among the earliest suggested applications of lasers were material processing such as cutting, drilling and welding, and applications in medicine. Initial results were quickly obtained by simple means. However, in order to optimize the procedure, and make it both reproducible and reliable, a knowledge of the interrelations between the primary action and subsequent secondary reactions was essential.

Medical laser applications are not only among those first suggested, but are also characterized by an unusual diversity that cuts across all medical disciplines. Nevertheless, a basic distinction can be made between diagnostic and therapeutic applications. In medical diagnosis, such properties of laser light as its monochromatism and coherence are exploited.

The small divergence of laser light and the resulting possibility of concentrating very high light intensity at the focal point of a lens are of decisive importance in therapy, with the exception of laser stimulation therapy. All applications in surgery and allied fields are based on the conversion of laser light into heat in tissue and the resulting thermal interactions.

Biophysical Relationships

An essential feature in the medical application of lasers is the action of laser radiation on biological molecules. In any consideration of the interaction between laser radiation and biological molecules (cells and tissues), the relationship between the physical parameters of the biological objects and the parameters of the laser radiation is important.

The thermal denaturation of tissue takes place roughly as follows. To a large extent both the structure and the function of living cells are determined by a wide variety of proteins. These macromolecules have a highly ordered structure which is energetically stable at body temperature. If the temperature is raised locally to about 50 °C or more, a certain percentage of the molecules pass into an energetically activated state from which an irreversible transition into the denaturated state takes place. When this happens, the protein molecule to some extent loses its spatial arrangement and thus its power to function in the cell. It should be noted that, irrespective of the nature of the irradiated tissue, individual thermolabile enzymes may play a leading part in the tissue reaction. There then follows a delayed tissue necrosis, although little or no structural damage to the tissue can be seen immediately after the irradiation.

Our knowledge of these physical and chemical cell and tissue parameters, of their influence on the primary interaction with laser radiation, and also of the physical and biological secondary reactions is still very incomplete. However, we know for certain that degree and extent of the thermal action depend both on the optical and thermal properties of the tissue and on the laser beam geometry and energy of the incident light.

The most important optical parameter is the wavelength-dependent absorption of biological molecules. Since the building blocks of living systems, amino acids, proteins, and nucleic acids are, despite their great variety, made up of only a few basic elements, a few fundamental rules can be formulated for the absorption of optical radiation. The main absorption of biological molecules occurs with wavelengths shorter than about 280 nm. At present there are only a few, mainly low-power lasers operating in this range of very strong absorption. The great majority of molecule-specific vibrational and rotational absorption bands are all in the range of wavelengths longer than 1,000 nm. With a few exceptions, optical radiation in the visible region is, therefore, hardly absorbed by biological objects. One of the most important exceptions to this rule is the hemoglobin in the red blood corpuscles and melanin which is stored as a pigment in the skin and also in large quantities in the pigment cells of the retina. Here, the absorption coefficient is particularly high in the green region of the spectrum.

The high water content of most tissue results in a very strong absorption of infrared radiation. Thus the absorption coefficient of tissue at 1,064 nm, the wavelength of the neodymium-YAG (Nd:YAG) laser, is typically about 10 cm^{-1}; at 10,600 nm, the wavelength of the CO_2 laser, it is about 200–1,000 cm^{-1}. This high absorption by water results in very efficient energy transfer and heating of the tissue during irradiation with laser beams of these wavelengths.

In addition to absorption, scattering must be considered a further optical tissue parameter. Tissue is a highly structured medium, so that directed optical radiation is completely altered in its spatial distribution as a result of, for example, reflection, refraction, and diffraction. This scattering effect is of importance mainly when absorption is weak.

The thermal properties of tissue, especially heat capacity and conductivity, may, to the first approximation, be assumed to be the same as those of water. However, estimation of the spread of the energy by thermal conductivitiy is often very difficult when tissue layers of strongly differing structure and complicated geometry are involved, such as the stomach wall, the retina, and the bladder wall, or when blood vessels result in a very nonhomogeneous removal of energy owing to the fact that the blood flow usually varies with time.

In addition, phase transitions such as evaporation or carbonization often occur during irradiation and considerably alter the optical and thermal properties of the tissue.

As can be seen, even the processes involved in the purely thermal interaction between laser radiation and biological tissue are highly complex. This makes it difficult to develop interaction models suitable for determining the optimal laser parameters for the purpose required, the most favorable irradiation geometry, and for predicting, at least qualitatively, the results to be expected. However, a consideration of the dependence of absorption and scattering in the tissue on wavelength alone permits a simple explanation of the various thermal effects of laser systems used in surgery [1–3].

Various Effects of Laser Radiation on the Tissue

The absorption of light in biological tissue, and thus also scattering, depends very strongly on the wavelength of the incident radiation. Because of the different proportions of absorption and scattering in the extinction of laser radiation in the tissue or, to put it differently, because of the different ratios of the absorption coefficient to the scattering coefficient, the various lasers used in surgery – the CO_2, the argon, and the Nd:YAG laser – differ with respect to their thermal penetration.

Action of CO_2 Laser Radiation on Bladder Tissue

With the CO_2 laser, which emits light in the middle infrared range (10,600 nm), absorption by the tissue is the strongest, and scattering is negligible. The light energy is, therefore, completely converted into heat at the tissue surface. For this reason the CO_2 laser, with its small depth of penetration, is well suited as a cutting tool for removing tissue.

At power outputs of 5–10 W the following process is observed on irradiation of bladder tissue with the CO_2 laser: First, rapid heating of the irradiated bladder section to above 100 °C occurs, leading to evaporation, carbonization, and rapid removal of the topmost layer of tissue. Only slight warming occurs beneath the surface. The result is a cutting effect due to the surface absorption of energy. The radiation is completely absorbed within a layer which is only 0.1–0.2 mm deep.

Action of Argon Laser Radiation on Bladder Tissue

The absorption of argon laser radiation, visible green light (495, 515 nm), is weaker than that of the CO_2 laser radiation, but stronger than that of the Nd:YAG laser. The scattering of the argon laser emission is, therefore, less pronounced during heating than that of the Nd:YAG laser, and the thermal penetration is smaller. The application of the argon laser is thus restricted to indications where removal of the tissue with simultaneous limited coagulation is desired.

When a bladder wall is irradiated with the argon laser at a power output of 4–8 W, a reaction similar to that seen with the CO_2 laser is observed. The removal effect at the surface, however, clearly depends on the dose of the radiation. After irradiation of the bladder surface with the argon laser at only 5 W for 2 s, a small tissue-removing effect is seen. The depth of the necrosis is about 0.5 mm. The adjacent connective tissue is thickened. Bundles of smooth wall muscle fibers close to the surface are included in the necrosis; the deeper wall layers are unchanged. When the dose is increased, the coagulation necrosis does not extend into the deeper layers of the bladder wall, but a crater-shaped tissue defect is produced, at the edge of which little carbonized material is deposited. The tissue-removing effect increases upon a further elevation of the energy density and ultimately leads to perforation.

Action of the Nd:YAG Laser Radiation on Bladder Tissue

The Nd:YAG laser emits light in the near infrared range (1,064 nm). Here, absorption in the tissue is very low. The optical scattering manifests itself strongly and promotes a uniform distribution of the radiation within the tissue. Owing to thermal penetration, the Nd:YAG laser is suitable for use as a coagulator whenever the aims are thermal denaturation without removal of tissue and little mechanical damage to the tissue surface.

When the Nd:YAG laser is used at a power of 40 W and an irradiation time of about 5 s, the process occurring in the bladder wall is different. Slow heating of a larger volume of tissue takes place around the target zone, followed by deep, slowly progressing coagulation; finally, the tissue water at the surface evaporates, resulting in evident shrinkage, although only a little of the surface tissue is destroyed. The surface is covered with a thin layer of fibrin. After Nd:YAG laser irradiation a band-shaped, deep-reaching coagulation necrosis is revealed, extending to all layers of the bladder wall down to the serosa with no primary tissue removal. Depending on the dosage applied, the coagulation depth is 2–6 mm [4, 5].

Surface cooling during irradiation has a strong influence on type and extent of tissue damage. With gas cooling irradiation produces a clearly demarcated necrosis on the tissue surface. The maximum coagulation depth with gas cooling or in air is about 4–5 mm; this can be increased to 5–6 mm, using liquid cooling. Tissue damage at the surface is then minimal, and the necrosis is almost drop shaped.

The coagulation volume initially increases with the energy density, but is then limited by backscattering from the blanched surface. If carbonization occurs at the surface, absorption is increased, and the tissue is vaporized. If the surface is cooled with a flow of liquid the onset of blanching is delayed. This prevents carbonization which leads to deep coagulation. One of the major advantages of the Nd:YAG laser is its ability to coagulate without vaporizing [6].

Also, a comparison between Nd:YAG laser coagulation and electrocoagulation is very interesting. Independently of the tissue structure, the thermal energy is distributed equally with Nd:YAG laser irradiation. The result is a clearly demarcated necrosis with a predictable and controllable depth of penetration [7, 8].

Owing to the deep penetrating effect of more than 5 mm, depending on the type of tissue and the dosage, the Nd:YAG laser acts like a coagulating instrument. The deep penetration and the broad damage zone of more than 5 mm make the sealing of blood vessels and lymph vessels possible [9].

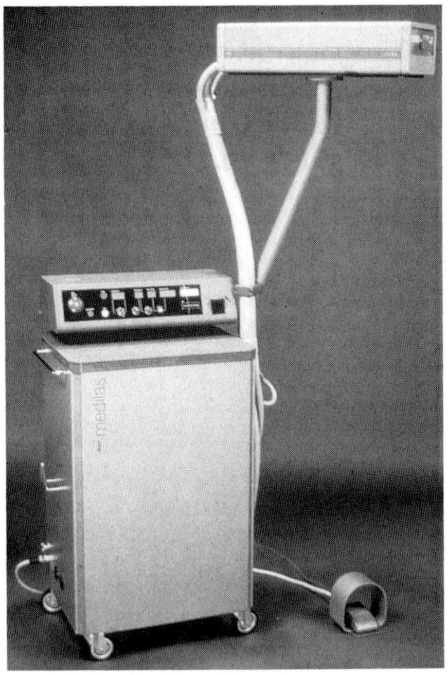
1

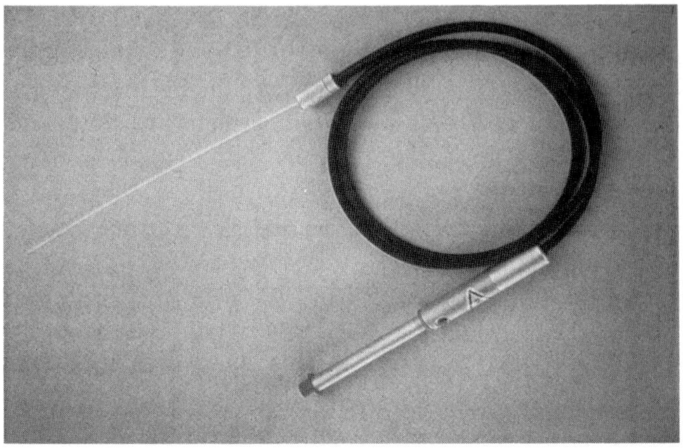

2

Fig. 1. Clinical Nd:YAG system mediLas 2 (manufacturer: MBB-Medizintechnik GmbH).

Fig. 2. Light guide system with liquid rinsing (manufacturer: MBB-Medizintechnik GmbH).

Description of the mediLas-YAG System

As an example of a medical Nd:YAG laser, the mediLas system is presented here along with various application instruments that are necessary for an efficient use of the laser.

The laser system comprises a mobile unit housing the power supply, the control unit, the cooling system, an operating console, and the laser head. The console permits digital selection of power and duration of the pulse. Power meter and power indicator unit are integrated. A printer records the indicated data for each laser pulse. The mains unit contains all the electrical supply elements. Electronic switching and monitoring elements render the system largely automatic. Mains water is used for the cooling system which is safeguarded by flow monitors and magnetic valves.

The system fulfils all requirements for clinical applications, i.e., it is simple to operate, small in size, and highly mobile. The safety features comply with the national and international safety regulations (fig. 1).

The laser head accommodates all the optical components of a Nd:YAG laser, i.e., the crystal, the pump lamps, the resonator mirrors, and the lamp housing together with a low-power pilot laser which emits light in the visible range. The pilot light is concentric with the therapeutic Nd:YAG beam. A helium-neon laser with a power of 1 mW is used for this purpose. Both radiations are jointly transmitted to the operation site by a flexible fiberoptic light guide. In this way the pilot light marks the target point for the therapeutic beam.

The transmission of the laser beam along flexible light guides depends upon total reflection at the interface of two media with different refractive indices. Light propagation takes place in the optically denser medium. The light wave travels from one end of the guide to the other via successive total reflections. The transmission takes place in quartz glass fibers.

Commercially available quartz optical fibers with a strong Teflon covering (fiber diameter 0.2–0.6 mm) fulfil all the requirements relating to mechanical stability and high flexibility. The transmission efficiency of this fiber system is 90%. The exit divergence of about 8° can be compensated by adjusting the irradiation distance and the use of appropriate lenses.

The light guide systems for rigid endoscopes are protected by metal-plastic tubes. The actual fiber can be passed through the endoscope. The light guides are attached to the laser head by means of a connector which incorporates the optical coupling system [10]. Such laser light guide systems are used with liquid rinsing in urological endoscopes (fig. 2).

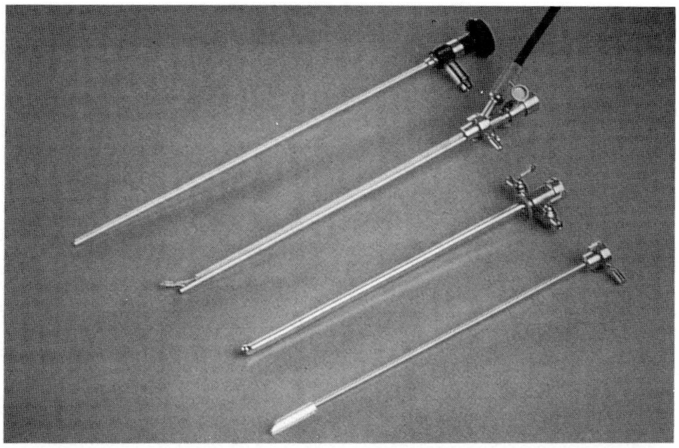
3

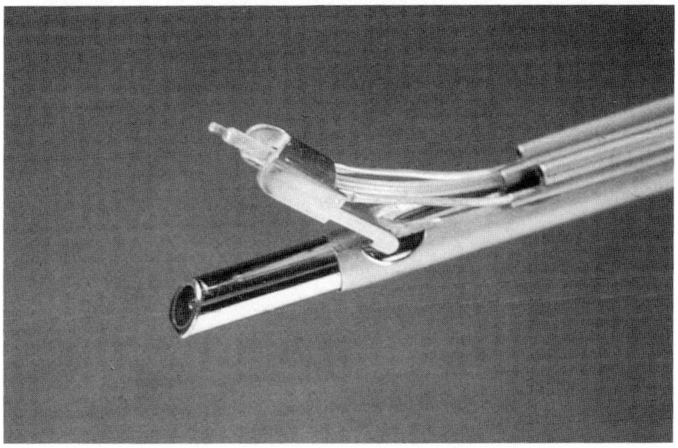
4

Fig. 3, 4. Laser cystoscope attachment with 21-french Albarran insert (manufacturer: Karl Storz GmbH & Co.).

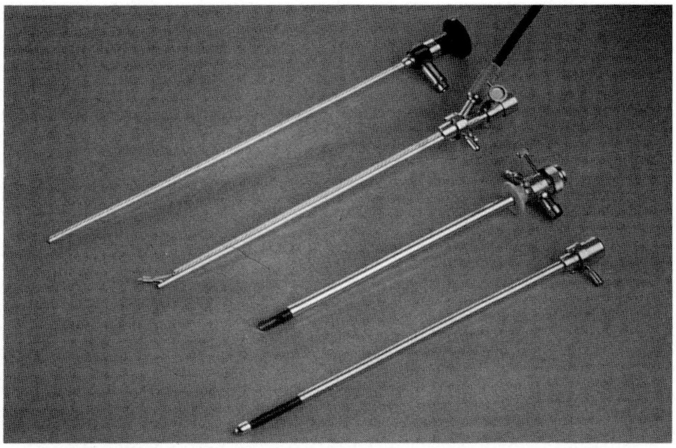
5

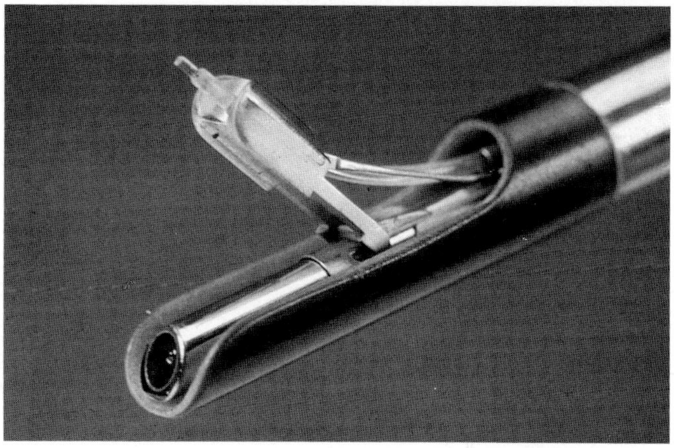
6

Fig. 5, 6. Laser cystoscope attachment with Albarran insert and 24-french resection sheath (manufacturer: Karl Storz GmbH & Co.).

Endoscopic Application

Suitable cystoscope attachments had to be developed for the transurethral use of laser beams in urology. For outpatients with small stage TIS and Tl bladder tumors, the instrument consists of a conventional urethrocystoscope sheath of 19- to 21-french (diameter 6–7 mm) standard inspection optics with variable viewing angles and a special laser cystoscope attachment. The light guide is passed through the ureteral catheter channel of an Albarran instrument [11, 12].

The distal end of the light guide can be flexed through an angle of up to about 80° using the Albarran lever which is designed to protect the end of the fiber. The end of the fiber can be moved axially be means of a spring system, so that the distance to the irradiation zone can be adjusted accurately (fig. 3, 4).

Water is introduced into the attachment and led to the distal end, so that with circulating rinsing the state of filling can easily be kept constant. Practically all regions of the bladder can be irradiated perpendicularly with this endoscopic system.

For clinical interventions on larger tumors and for laser irradiation of the tumor bed after electroresection, a 24-french resection sheath with an oblique tip and a central cock is used instead of the sheath described above. The greater rinsing effect that can be achieved with this arrangement permits efficient laser beam irradiation, even when bleeding occurs (fig. 5, 6).

For interventions within the urethra in the treatment of urethral carcinomas and condylomas, a system with a 20-french sheath and an additional overall reflux sheath can be used. In this case there is no need for the Albarran lever, since the fiber is passed directly through the laser

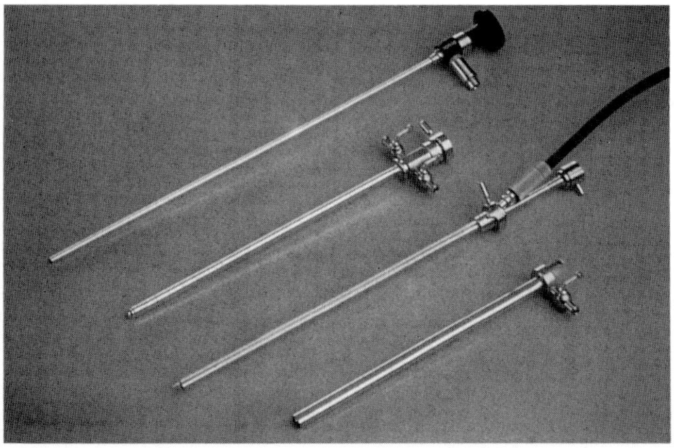

7

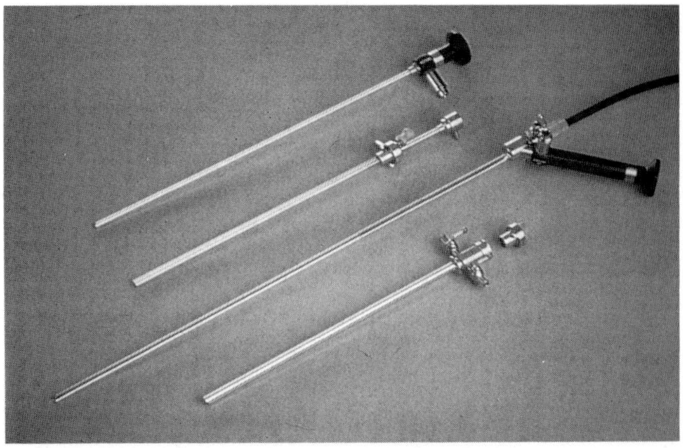

9

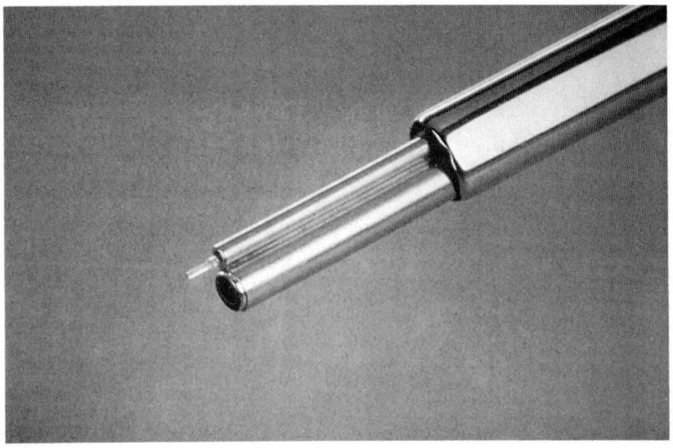

8

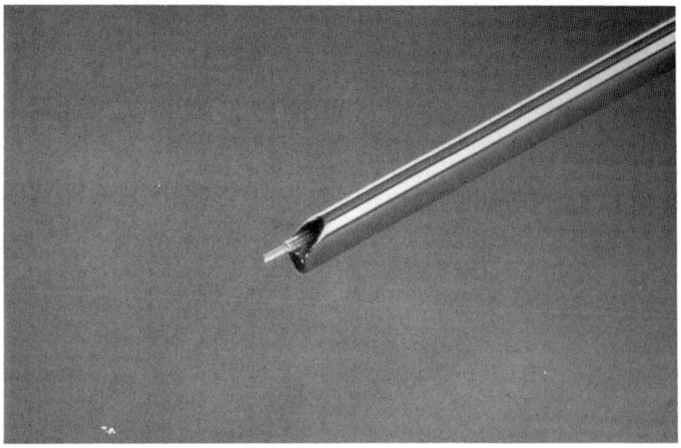

10

Fig. 7, 8. Laser urethroscope with 20-french overall reflux sheath (manufacturer: Karl Storz GmbH & Co.).

Fig. 9, 10. Laser ureterorenoscope 9-french and inspection insert (manufacturer: Karl Storz GmbH & Co.).

insert together with the inspection optic [13]. Any damage that might possibly be done to the urethral mucosa by the Albarran instrument is thus avoided (fig. 7, 8).

A 9-french ureterorenoscope has been designed for tumor treatment within the lower part of the ureter. An inspection insert, with a bougie channel, facilitates the introduction of the instrument. Fiber and viewing optic are inserted into the part of the system which will be passed into the ureter (fig. 9, 10).

For the irradiation of tumors in the pelvis and the calices of the kidney a special flexible endoscope with a lumen of only 4 mm can be used. The light guide and rinsing fluid are passed through the working channel (fig. 11, 12).

Applications in Open Surgery

For all operations on an exposed area or for external applications, various operation handpieces have been designed [14]. The focusing handpiece utilizes an interchangeable optic. Focal points down to 0.4 mm in diameter can be achieved. By altering the irradiation distance, power density and diameter of the treated area can be varied (fig. 13).

For open interventions where surface cooling is necessary to achieve deep necrosis without surface damage, simple hand applicators of different shapes have been designed. The slim configuration of the instrument ensures unimpaired vision for unrestricted, free-hand manipulation, in particular when they are used under the microscope (fig. 14).

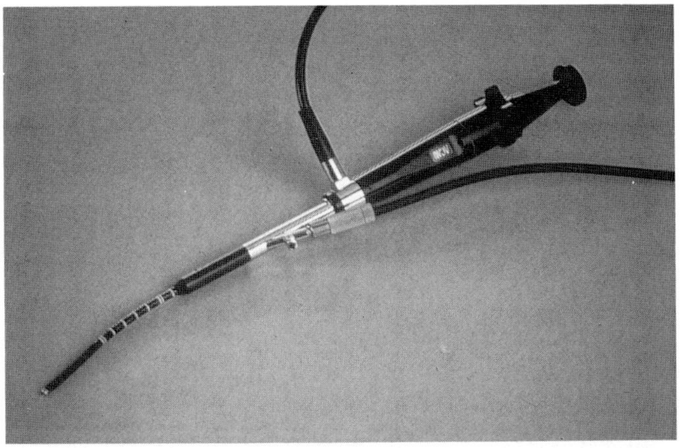

1

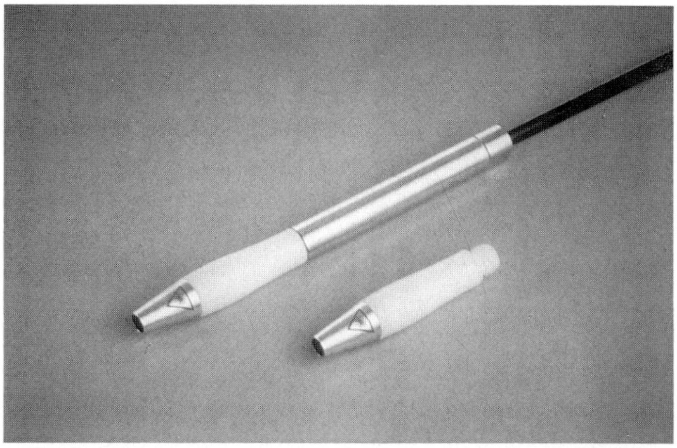

13

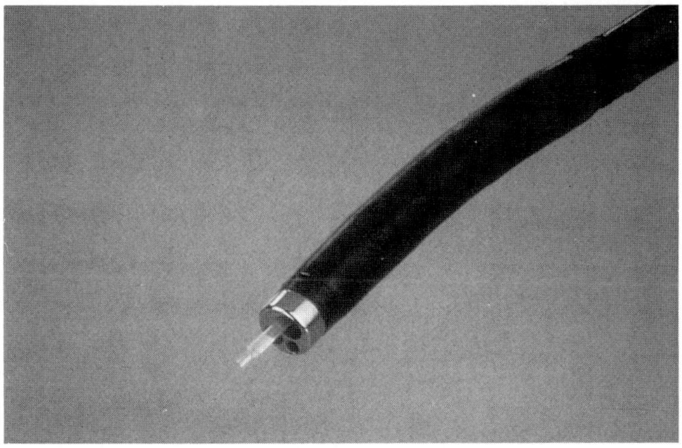

2

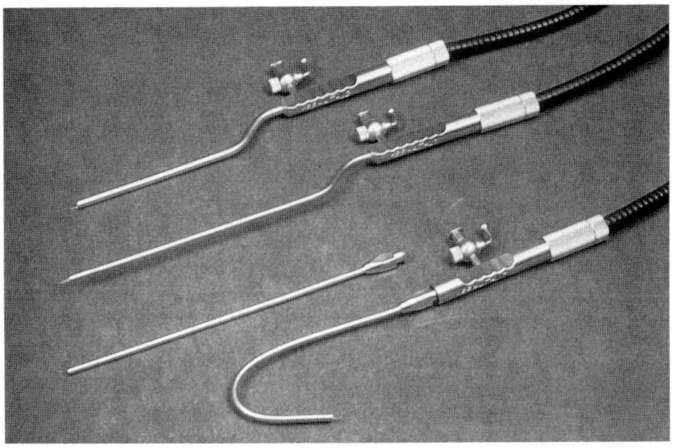

14

Fig. 11, 12. Flexible nephroscope with laser light guide, outside diameter 4.6 mm (manufacturer: ACMI, Inc.).

Fig. 13. Focusing handpiece with interchangeable optic (manufacturer: MBB-Medizintechnik GmbH).

Fig. 14. Hand applicators with liquid-protected light guide (manufacturer: MBB-Medizintechnik GmbH).

Safety Aspects

The prerequisite for the use of high-power lasers for surgical interventions in medicine is complete safety for the patient, the doctor, and auxiliary personnel with respect to laser radiation hazards. The aim of clinical laser therapy is to achieve controlled denaturation of organic tissue. The laser radiation at the site of the treatment must be of sufficient intensity to produce the desired thermal action. However, at the same time it is essential to ensure that the radiation intensity outside the treatment region is limited, so that there is no risk to the doctor or his assistants. Moreover, there must be adequate protection against any radiation unintentionally emitted outside the operating field.

Eye hazards are by far the most important. Various structures of the eye may be injured, depending upon which structure absorbs the greatest radiant energy per volume of tissue. In the case of lasers emitting light in the visible and near infrared region between 400 and 1,400 nm, such as the Nd:YAG laser, the main danger is retinal damage because of the transparency of the lens of the eye.

If the laser beam is reflected, it is the nature of the reflection that is important. Diffuse reflections are generally not hazardous, except with high-power laser beams. Directed reflections are dangerous, since the small divergence of the laser beam is retained.

The most unfavorable case is when the parallel laser light is focused on the smallest possible spot on the retina.

A beam of 50 W/m^2 at the cornea becomes one of 25 MW/m^2 on the retina.

The use of the Nd:YAG laser in endoscopic and open surgery necessitates a number of different safety precautions corresponding to the different techniques and irradiation parameters. Various endoscopes and several handpieces have been experimentally tested in order to measure the radiation exposure to the eye caused by backscattering. The information gained has been compared with the MPE values defined in the draft of the International Electrotechnical Commission. The irradiation parameters were varied in accordance with the clinical procedure. When using the rigid laser cystoscopes, in the worst possible case, e.g., at a viewing distance of 8 mm, an irradiation distance of 3 mm and an output power of 50 W, the radiation exposure is still appreciably below the MPE value.

In the case of the tested flexible system, especially with an exposure time longer than 0.5 s, radiation exposure values that are above the permissible level occur. For this reason the eyepiece should always be fitted with a filter such as the KG 3 Schott filter of 2 mm thickness with a transmission coefficient of 10^{-3} for the Nd:YAG laser wavelength.

For interventions with the surgical handpiece in which the surgeon has a visual distance of about 25 cm, the radiation exposure limit for the eye is exceeded by a considerable margin, even with an initial laser output of 50 W. Although the exposure to backscattered radiation at a distance of 1 m is certainly below the MPE value, direct radiation can escape into the operation room, especially when the handpiece is used without due care. Thus, all the people present at the operation must wear protective glasses. Adequate protective glasses, in accordance with safety regulations, are commercially available (i.e. Germany: DIN 582I5 Schutzklasse LGA).

Provided that the laser is properly used, the protective effect of the recommended filters and protective glasses is sufficient to avoid accidents. However, in particular in the case of endoscopic operations, it should be noted that the laser beam should not be triggered until the laser endoscope has been inserted into the stomach or bladder or any other organ concerned. The opportunity for free manipulation offered by the surgical handpiece calls for special care, and protective glasses should always be worn.

Moreover, for complete patient safety it is necessary to determine the optimal irradiation dose. The irradiation dose is optimal when the tumors infiltrating the bladder wall are totally destroyed by heat without the neighboring organs being damaged. Accordingly, a bladder wall tumor extending to a depth of 4 mm can be adequately treated with a laser power of 45 W and an exposure time of 2–4 s. A normal bladder wall thickness suffices to protect the adjacent intestinal loops from the transmitted radiation [16–19].

On the basis of the experience of the last 10 years, it has been shown that proper application of the mediLas YAG laser equipment, compliance with the recommended safety precautions, and the use of a dose appropriate to the medical indication ensure complete safety for patient, surgeon, and clinical personnel.

References

1 Hofstetter, A.; Frank, F.: The neodymium-YAG laser in urology (Hoffmann-La Roche, Basel 1980).

2 Halldorsson, Th.: Biophysikalische und apparative Grundlagen der endovesikalen Nd:YAG-Laserapplikation. Urologe A *20:* 291–299 (1981).

3 Frank, F.; Hofstetter, A.; Keiditsch, E.: Experimental investigations and new instrumentation for Nd:YAG laser treatment in urology; in Bellina, Gynecologic laser surgery, pp. 345–356 (Plenum Publishing, New York 1981).

4 Frank, F.; Hofstetter, A.; Böwering, R.; Keiditsch, E.: Endoscopic application of the Nd:YAG laser in urology. Biophysical fundamentals and instrumentation. Proc. Soc. photo-opt. Inst. Eng. *211:* 36–40 (1979).

5 Hofstetter, A.: Endoskopische Zerstörung von Blasentumoren mit Laser. Urologe A *20:* 317–322 (1981).

6 Landthaler, M.; Brunner, R.; Haina, D.; Frank, F.; Waidelich, W.; Braun-Falco, O.: Neodym-YAG-Laser in der Dermatologie. MMW *126:* 1108–1112 (1984).

7 Keiditsch, E.; Hofstetter, A.; Rothenberger, K.; Maiwald, H.; Stern, J.; Pensel, J.; Frank, F.: Comparative morphological investigations of the effects of the neodym-YAG laser and electrocoagulation in experimental animal research; in Bellina, Gynecologic laser surgery, pp. 327–336 (Plenum Publishing, New York 1981).

8 Keiditsch, E.: Histologische Grundlagen der endovesikalen Neodym-YAG-Laserbestrahlung. Urologe A *20:* 293–300 (1981).

9 Zimmermann, I.; Stern, J.; Frank, F.; Keiditsch, E.; Hofstetter, A.: Interception of lymphatic drainage by Nd:YAG laser irradiation in rat urinary bladder. Lasers Surg. Med. *4:* 167–172 (1984).

10 Frank, F.; Bailer, P.; Beck, O.; Böwering, R.; Hofstetter, A.: Instrumentation for the surgical application of the Nd:YAG laser. Proc. Soc. photo-opt. Inst. Eng. *405:* 105–109 (1984).

11 Hofstetter, A.; Frank, F.: Ein neues Laser-Endoskop zur Bestrahlung von Blasentumoren. Fortschr. Med. *97:* 232–234 (1979).

12 Hofstetter, A.; Frank, F.; Keiditsch, E.; Böwering, R.: Endoscopic neodymium-YAG laser application for destroying bladder tumors. Eur. Urol. *7:* 278–282 (1981).

13 Hofstetter, A.; Böwering, R.; Keiditsch, E.; Frank, F.: Zerstörung von Uretertumoren mit dem Neodym-YAG-Laser. Fortschr. Med. *101:* 625–627 (1983).

14 Staehler, G.: Die externe Applikation von Neodym-YAG-Laserstrahlen in der Urologie. Urologe A *20:* 323–327 (1981).
15 Frank, F.; Halldorsson, Th.: Untersuchungen zur Sicherheit bei der klinischen Anwendung des Neodym-YAG-Lasers. Medsche Physik *1981:* 723–727.
16 Pensel, J.; Hofstetter, A.; Frank, F.; Keiditsch, E.; Rothenberger, K.: Temporal and spatial temperature profile of the bladder serosa in intravesical neodymium-YAG-laser irradiation. Eur. Urol. *7:* 298–303 (1981).
17 Rothenberger, K.; Pensel, J.; Hofstetter, A.; Keiditsch, E.; Stern, J.: Dosierung der Neodym-YAG-Laserbestrahlung zur endovesikalen Anwendung bei Blasentumoren: tierexperimentelle Untersuchungen. Urologe A *20:* 310–314 (1981).
18 Hofstetter, A.; Schmiedt, E.; Staehler, G.: Endovesikale Zerstörung von Blasentumoren mit dem Neodym-YAG-Laser. Urologe A *21:* 9–11 (1982).
19 Staehler, G.; Halldorsson, T.; Langerholc, J.; Bilgram. R.: Dosimetry for neodymium:YAG applications in urology. Lasers Surg. Med. *1:* 191–197 (1980).

Dr. F. Frank,
MBB-Medizintechnik GmbH,
Postfach 80 11 68,
D–8000 München 80 (FRG)

Eur. Urol. 12: suppl. 1, pp. 12–16 (1986)

Morphological Fundamentals in the Treatment of Tumors with the Neodymium-YAG Laser

E. Keiditsch

Institut für Pathologie, Klinikum München-Bogenhausen, München, BRD

Key Words. Neodymium-YAG laser · Sealing of lymphatics · Urinary bladder tumors

Abstract. On the basis of experimental animal research regarding type, distribution, and depth of necrosis in urinary bladder under neodymium-YAG (Nd:YAG) laser irradiation, identical results have been confirmed in human tissue. Bladder tumors indicated for cystectomy have first been treated with the Nd:YAG laser and histologically examined. Destruction of tumor tissue is demonstrated. Particular attention was paid to the temporary closing of the lymphatic drainage system due to the deep coagulation capability of the Nd:YAG laser irradiation. Nd:YAG laser irradiation is especially suitable for tumor coagulation, since simultaneous interception of lymphatic drainage will inhibit the spreading of tumor cells.

The possibility of transmission of laser light via flexible light guides, the development and constant improvement of the instrumentarium required for endoscopic application, and, last but not least, its excellent coagulation properties have created for the neodymium-YAG (Nd:YAG) laser a permanent niche in endoscopic and open treatment of tumors in the field of urology. At the same time, the field of application of the Nd:YAG laser used as described, has increasingly expanded to cover other specialities, e.g., pulmonology, gastroenterology, dermatology, and others.

If, under experimental conditions, depth and extent of necroses developing after conventional electrocoagulation and laser coagulation [1, 2] are compared in homogeneous liver tissue, differences are found merely in the extension into the depths, while, in the multilayered tissue of the urinary bladder, the results obtained vary (fig. 1): unsharply delimited, irregular, and predominantly superficial necroses are found after electrocoagulation in contrast to deep, sharply delimited necroses after laser coagulation.

Both forms of necrosis – after electrocoagulation and after laser coagulation – represent thermal coagulation necroses which, qualitatively, cannot be unequivocally differentiated from one another. There are, however, clear differences with respect to 'arrangement' and extension. Electrocoagulation leads to a thermal necrosis, the extent of which, both laterally in the surface and also into the depths, is *not* predictable. Since with respect to high-frequency applications, biological tissue behaves like an ohmic resistance, the electrical conductivity depends upon the nature of the tissue. Thus, the specific resistance of such vascular tissue as muscle is relatively low, while that of fatty tissue is considerably higher – by a factor of about 20. This explains why the high-frequency currents spread where the resistance is smallest, e.g., over the surface or also along the blood vessels. In contrast to the necrosis induced by electrocoagulation, laser necrosis leads to a *reproducible* uniformly ribbon-like, and thus *controllable,* necrosis with sharply delimited margins and complete destruction of the tissue down to a depth of 4 mm – a point that is of great importance for the treatment of tumors of the bladder, the walls of which have a thickness of 4–5 mm. A decisive factor, however, is the fact that the pre-existing wall structure, comprising necrotic muscle fiber and collagen fiber structures, together with the elastic fibers, remains intact, so that secondary perforation is avoided [3]. Furthermore, the deep ne-

1 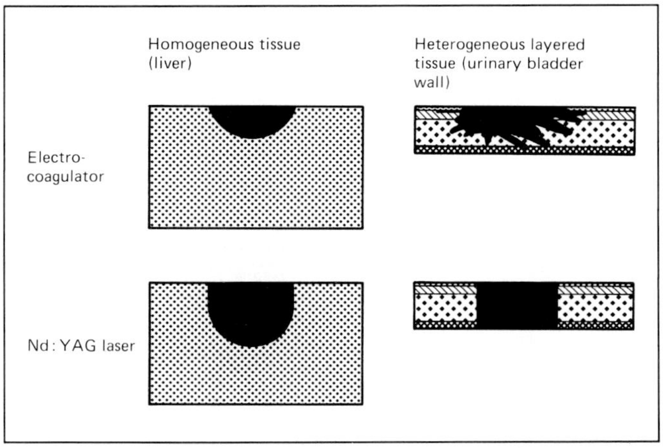

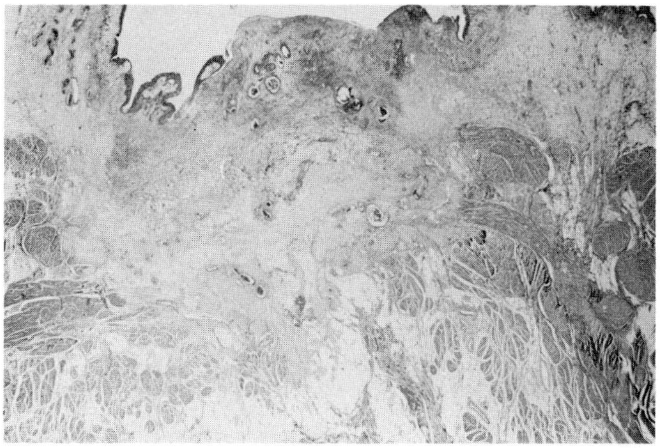 2

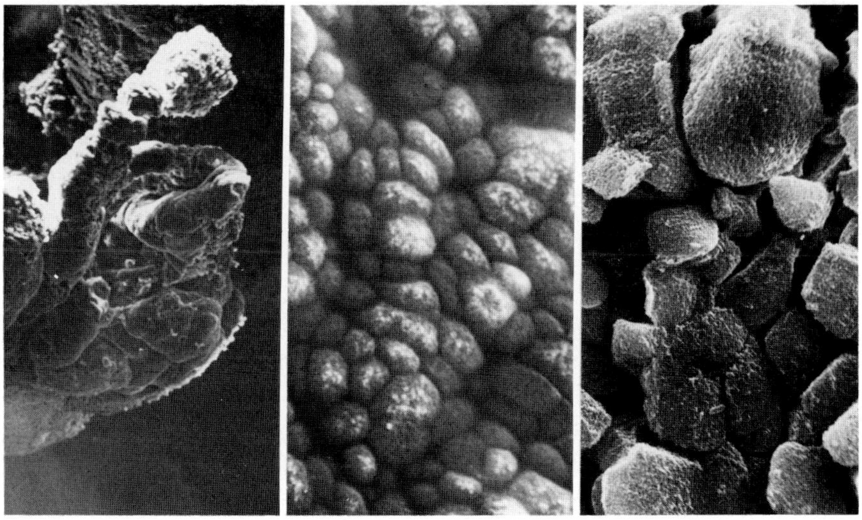 3

Fig. 1. Comparative schematic representation of the tissue damage following electrocoagulation and Nd:YAG laser irradiation as seen in liver tissue and in the multilayered wall of the bladder.

Fig. 2. Transmural Nd:YAG laser coagulation necrosis, laterally sharply demarcated by preserved smooth muscle fibers in human bladder (cystectomy specimen).

Fig. 3. Exophytic papillary carcinoma, the upper part of which has been coagulated by laser (left); undamaged surface epithelium (middle), and disorganization of the surface epithelium after laser coagulation (right).

croses, e.g., in the 'roof' (superior surface) of the bladder, are very rapidly covered from the serosal side by proliferation of mesenchymal structures.

These experimental results have also been confirmed in the human bladder. In patients scheduled for cystectomy, about 48 h prior to surgery, laser coagulation necroses were induced in the region of the tumor and the lesions subsequently investigated in the cystectomy specimen. A laterally sharply demarcated transmural necrosis extending, in the ideal case, into the subserosal fatty tissue was found (fig. 2), the depth of the necrosis decreasing with tangential irradiation or increased absorption of the laser light on carbonization of the tissue or in the presence of bleeding. In the irradiated region, the tumor tissue was completely destroyed, and after 2–3 days its margins were only vaguely discernible [4].

Irrespective of the various preinvasive neoplasias in the bladder, such as severe dysplasia, carcinoma in situ, or papillary carcinoma, the findings established in human bladders document the possibility and practicability of employing transmural laser coagulation to destroy even invasive carcinomas up to stage T_2 and, possibly, even T_{3a}.

Immediately after laser coagulation, the endoscopically blanched exophytic tumors reveal clearly discernible shrinkage artefacts of the surface relief when examined in the scanning electron microscope, as here in this example of a papillary tumor which reveals a 'grazing shot', as it were. In contrast to the normal urothelium, the coagulation zone reveals a disruption of the epithelium and escape of denatured erythrocytes (fig. 3). In particular, in the case of larger tumors that are partly covered

Table I. Regional lymph nodes of the rat urinary bladder marked by Indian ink

	Time, days											
	0	1	2	3	4	5	6	7	9	14	19	25
Control	+	+	+	+	+	+	++	++				
	0	++	+	+	+	+						
Laser	0	0	0	0	++	0	0					
	0	0	0	0	+	0						
	0	0	0	0	0	0	0	0	+	+	+	+

0 = Macroscopically and histologically negative.
+ = Histologically positive, macroscopically uncertain.
++ = Macroscopically positive.

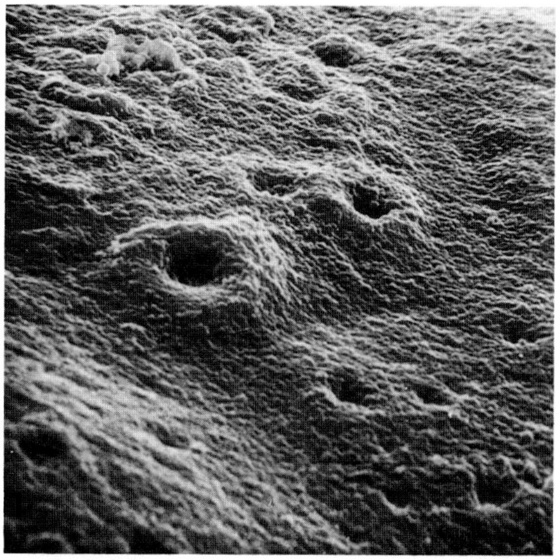

Fig. 4. Crater-like openings in the fibrin layer caused by escaping steam during laser coagulation.

with fibrin, crater-like openings are to be found in the fibrin layer – the result of escaping steam (fig. 4).

This disruption and dissociation of the surface epithelium is also very clearly recognizable under the light microscope, with separation of the urothelium, coagulation artefacts in the form of rod-like nuclei, and a usually edematous stroma (fig. 5). Despite marked thermal artefacts, relatively reliable grading is possible immediately after laser treatment, although, with increasing thermal effects including vaporization and carbonization, grading becomes less and less possible and may finally even be impossible. Of decisive importance is the optimal work-up of the biopsy material and an appropriate knowledge of the coagulation artefacts.

The coagulated exophytic tumor tissue very rapidly becomes necrotic, with complete desquamation of the surface epithelium, so that, already after 24 h, only necrotic stroma is to be seen. Such completely necrotic tumor rests can – if not sloughed – be of clinical importance, since during the process of reepithelialization they serve the newly forming epithelium as a 'bridge' and, usually 3–4 weeks after coagulation, can mimic a local recurrent lesion (fig. 6). Small newly formed structures appearing in the coagulation area relatively soon after laser coagulation should, therefore, not simply be subjected to follow-up coagulation, but should be excised in order, while avoiding coagulation artefacts, to differentiate such a pseudorecurrence from a true local reccurrence – a point that in the last analysis is of decisive importance for the statistical efficacy of laser coagulation with respect to local recurrence.

Since, as a rule, carcinomas of the bladder have a tendency to spread via the lymphatics, the question arises as to the extent to which lymph flow is influenced by laser coagulation. Decisive for the examination carried out to investigate this question was, on the one hand, the general idea of tumor seeding during the surgical intervention, e.g., on electroresection, and on the other hand, the freedom from recurrent disease of laser-coagulated patients (from earlier years) with invasive carcinomas and histologically demonstrated lymphangiosis carcinomatosa [5].

To this end we investigated the influence of transmural laser coagulation on lymph drainage from the urinary bladder of the rat (fig. 7) by injecting an intramural depot of water-insoluble Indian ink into the 'roof' of the bladder and observing the outflow of the ink along the parailiacal and paraaortic lymph nodes [6].

These experimental investigations have shown that transmural laser coagulation interrupts lymph flow for a period of 8 days. Not until the 9th day, i.e., later than recapillarization, do new lymph spaces form, so that deposited Indian ink can gradually be carried away (table I).

If the possibility of implantation of tumor cell complexes during a surgical intervention is the leading con-

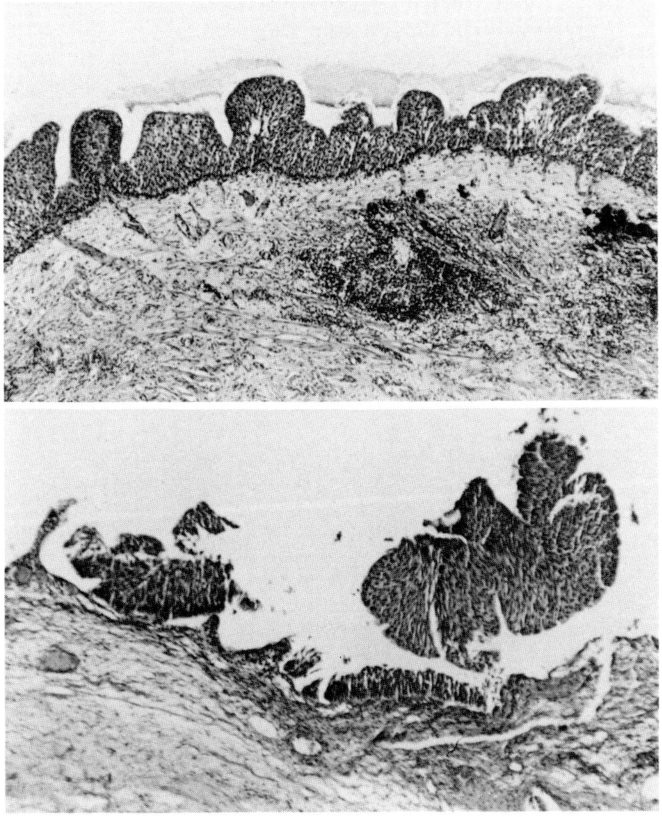

5

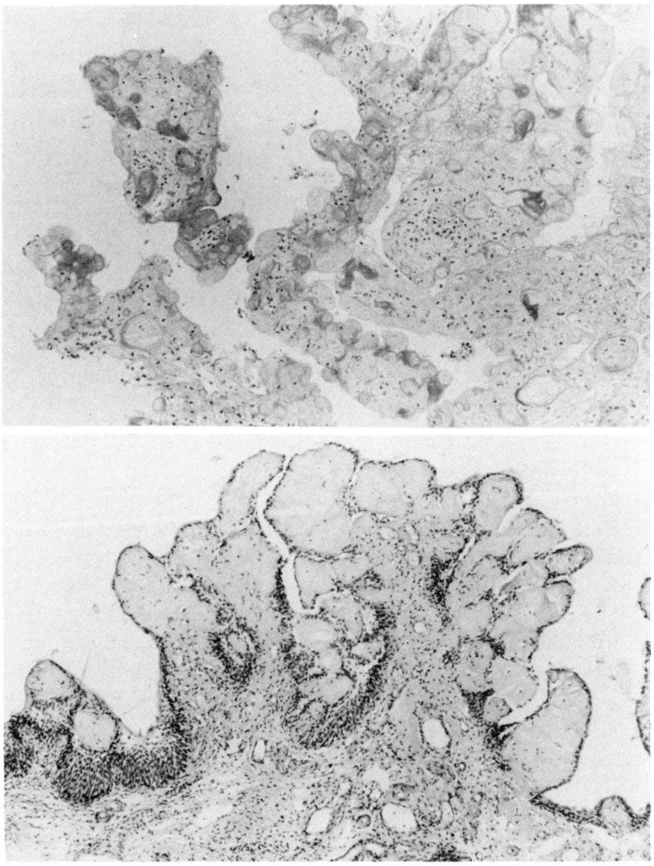

6

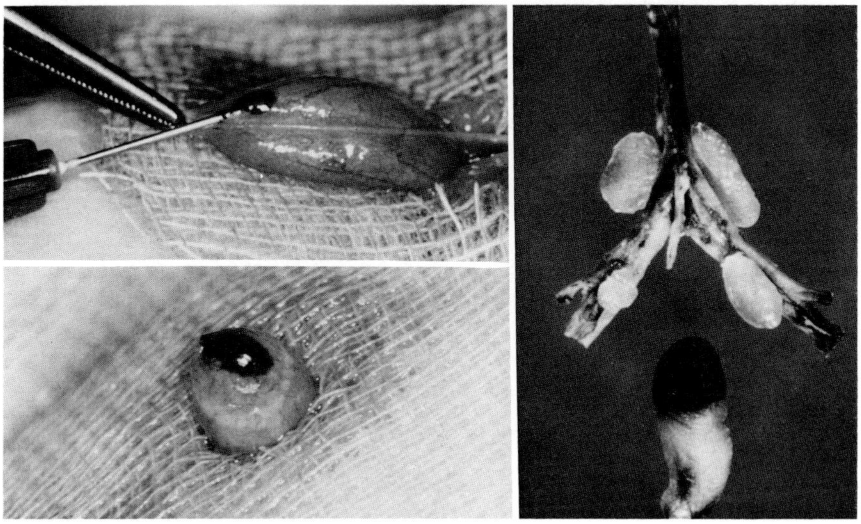

7

Fig. 5. Incipient papillary carcinoma of the bladder (G_1) before (above) and after (below) Nd:YAG laser irradiation.

Fig. 6. Necrotic tumor stroma portions (above) with complete desquamation of the epithelium and reepithelialization at the surface (below).

Fig. 7. Interruption of the lymph drainage after Nd:YAG laser coagulation. Implantation of the Indian ink (above, left); state after circular Nd:YAG laser coagulation (below, left), and interruption of the Indian ink flow off (right). The Indian ink marking does not exceed the laser marking. No staining of the parailiacal and para-aortic lymph nodes.

sideration, in particular with combined tumor treatment employing customary resection and laser coagulation of the tumor bed, experimental results suggest the need for a circular laser coagulation around the region of the tumor prior to resection. The results of the clinical studies carried out to date document more than merely a marked reduction in local recurrent lesions. An observation period of more than 4 years in still recurrence-free patients with histologically confirmed invasive carcinomas and demonstrated lymphangiosis carcinomatosa points to the effectiveness of laser therapy which, although in the last resort a thermal coagulation technique, is controllable and, with respect to its extension, in particular into the depths, both definable and reproducible. Whether the rigorous use of circular perifocal laser coagulation to avoid tumor seeding during the surgical intervention will improve the clinical results so far obtained remains to be seen.

Acknowledgement

The author is grateful to Dr.-Ing. H. Klingele, Munich, FRG, for performing the scanning electron microscopic examinations.

References

1 Keiditsch, E.: Histologische Grundlagen der endovesicalen Neodym-YAG-Laserbestrahlung. Urologe A *20:* 300–304 (1981).
2 Keiditsch, E.; Hofstetter, A.; Rothenberger, K.; Maiwald, H.; Stern, J.; Pensel, J.; Frank, F.: Comparative morphological investigations of the effects of the neodym-YAG laser and electrocoagulation in experimental animal research; in Bellina, Gynecologic laser surgery, pp. 327–336 (Plenum Publishing, New York 1981).
3 Keiditsch, E.; Langer, E.; Staehler, G.; Hofstetter, A.: Morphologische Veränderungen an der Kaninchenharnblase nach Laserbestrahlung. Verh. dt. Ges. Path. *61:* 367 (1977).
4 Keiditsch, E.; Hofstetter, A.; Zimmermann, I.; Stern, J.; Frank, F.; Babaryka, I.: Histological investigation to substantiate the therapy of bladder tumors with the neodymium-YAG laser. Laser *1:* 19–23 (1985).
5 Hofstetter, A.G.; Keiditsch, E.; Schmiedt, E.; Frank, F.: Der Neodym-YAG-Laser in der Urologie. Fortschr. Med. *102:* 885–890 (1984).
6 Zimmermann, I.; Stern, J.; Frank, F.; Keiditsch, E.; Hofstetter, A.: Interception of lymphatic drainage by Nd:YAG laser irradiation in rat urinary bladder. Lasers Surg. Med. *4:* 167–172 (1984).

Dr. E. Keiditsch,
Institut für Pathologie,
Klinikum München-Bogenhausen,
Postfach 86 05 96,
D–8000 München 86 (FRG)

Eur. Urol. *12:* suppl. 1, pp. 17–20 (1986)

0302–2838/86/0127–0017$2.75/0

Dosimetry of the Neodymium-YAG Laser in Urological Applications

J. Pensel

Department of Urology, Medical University of Lübeck, FRG

Key Words. Bladder tumors · Laser therapy · Dosimetry · Functional changes

Abstract. Animal experiments were carried out to optimize laser parameters for the treatment of superficial bladder tumors. The most important parameter affecting laser therapy is temperature. During intravesical irradiation of rabbit bladders, spatial and temporal temperature profiles on the bladder serosa were displayed. With these results adequate and safe treatment of bladder tumors is possible. We were unable to find any reduction in the hydrostatic capacity within the physiological range of bladder filling after laser irradiation of even 30% of the wall. Large diverticula developed within the first days after treatment, but had almost disappeared after 40 days.

With the growing use of lasers in medicine and surgery, more and more biophysical details of the interaction of the electromagnetic radiation with living tissue are becoming known. Intensive investigations have contributed much to the fact that laser therapy has become well known and safe. In particular, a knowledge of dosimetry and of corresponding histological changes permits optimal appliction of lasers in medicine.

The physical heterogeneity of biological tissue results in considerable regional variation in light absorption and scattering. These are two critical processes which determine the pattern of heating. The thermal effects of laser radiation caused by the interaction of infrared laser light with biological tissue have been studied widely [1–4]. The different biological effects of the various types of laser are explained by the very narrow range of laser light at defined regions of the spectrum. The effet of all types of laser is caused mainly by the heating of the tissue as a consequence of light absorption. Further biological effects are, to date, not well known.

In the case of the neodymium-YAG laser the biological tissue absorbs the light to a small extent, so that it can penetrate into deep layers and heat a large volume [3]. On heating the tisse up to 60 °C for several seconds, cytoglobulin is denatured [7, 8]. The cells, therefore, become necrotic, but the coarse structure is preserved, and there is only little reduction in mechanical stability of the tissue. In the region of the bladder wall there is no risk of perforation, even with transmural necroses, owing to the presence of fibers. Therefore, the neodymium-YAG laser is highly suitable for the treatment of bladder tumors [10].

An appropriate neodymium-YAG laser dose has to fulfill the following two requirements: (1) radical devitalization of the tumor as a whole and (2) no damage to neighboring organs (e.g., adjacent intestinal loops).

To comply with the first requirement, we have examined the temporal and spatial distribution of temperature on the outer wall of the urinary bladder in rabbits in relation to tissue thickness during intravesical neodymium-YAG laser irradiation [9]. The temperature at the outer wall helps to determine the laser parameters that allow for transmural necrosis. Figure 1 represents the isothermic temperature profile of the outer bladder wall during intravesical laser irradiation in the form of two pulses. The dotted zone indicates the radius of the directly irradiated wall area. Owing to the steep flanks of the temperature profile, the extent of heat-devitalized tissue is sharply limited. The effective diameter of the laser beam is determined primarily by the radiation profile of the scattered light. The influence of thermal diffusion is insignificant.

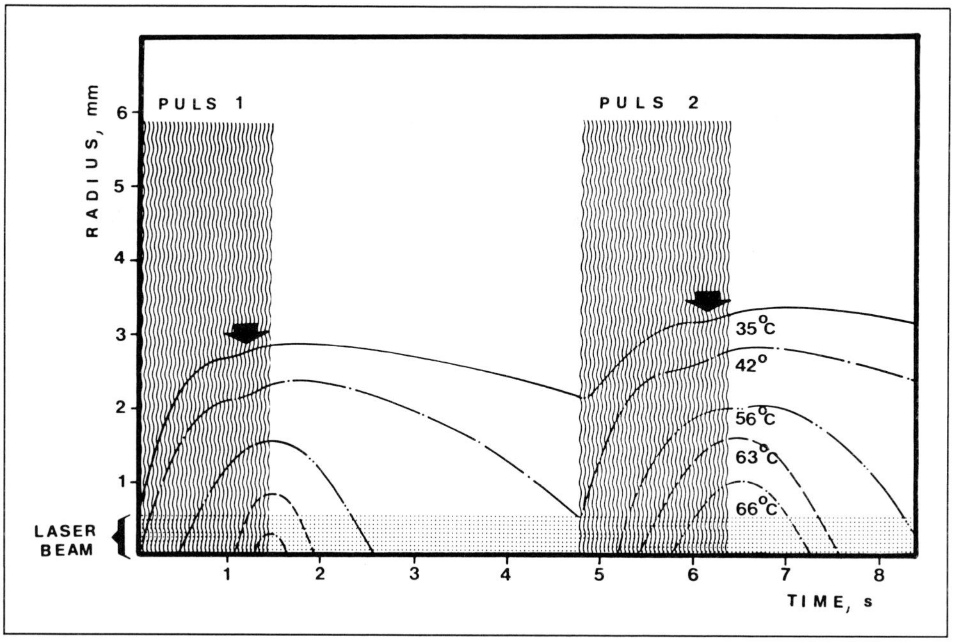

Fig. 1. Isothermal representation of the temperature profile of the outer bladder wall. Power density: 26 W·mm^{-2}; wall thickness: 2.3 mm; filling: NaCl solution.

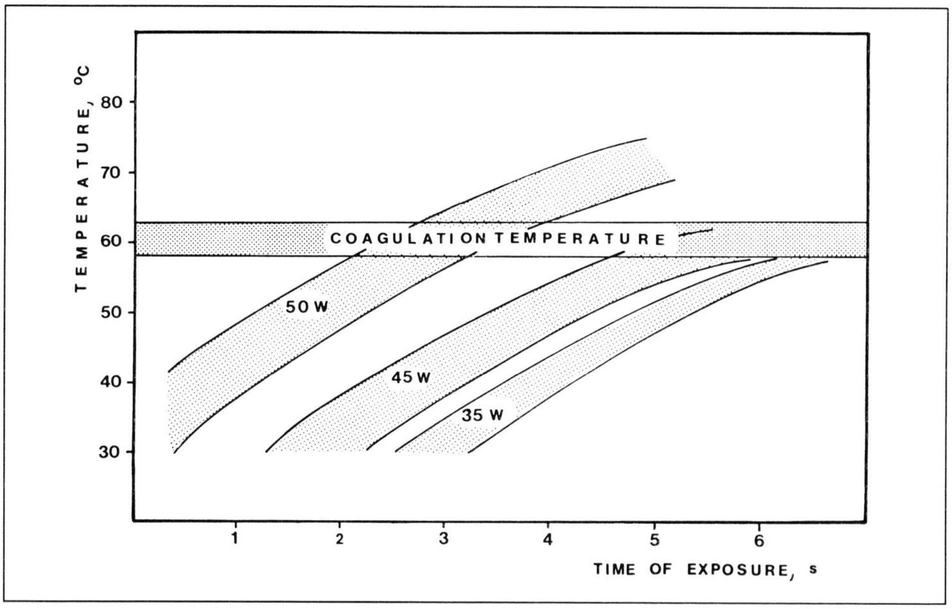

Fig. 2. Serosa temperature as a function of exposure time for three laser output powers. Wall thickness: 7 mm.

Thermal destruction of living tissue is an effect of both temperature and duration of heating, the two parameters having an integral correlation [8]. The experimental parameters were power density of the laser light, irradiation time, and bladder wall thickness. Assuming a basal tissue temperature of 30 °C and a wall thickness of 7 mm, the temperature profiles shown in figure 2 were obtained for three laser power levels. With a laser output power of 45 W, the therapeutic coagulation temperature of about 60 °C is reached only after an irradiation time of 5 s.

The temperature gradients can be used to estimate the temperature in the region of the irradiated tissue during the laser pulse. The cell destruction in turn correlates with this temperature, allowing prediction of the damage not to individual cells, but only to the whole tissue [5, 6]. The degree of coagulation depends on the temperature reached and on the duration of hyperthermia and can be estimated using the Arrhenius integral [8].

Variations in irradiation time are relatively noncritical. The light scattered in the irradiated tissue volume

3
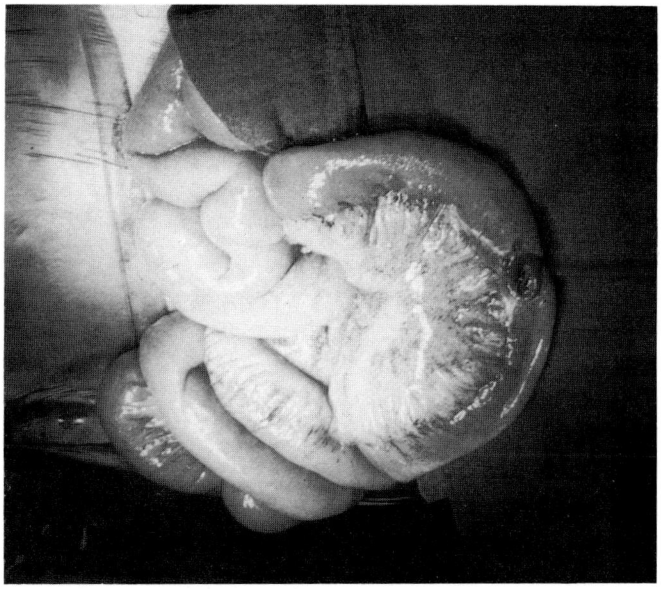

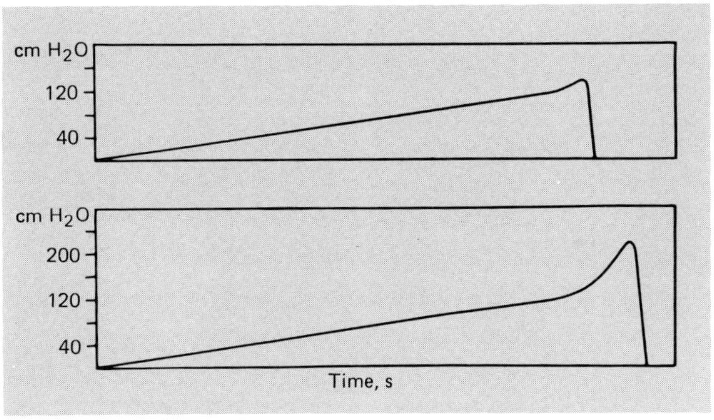

4

Fig. 3. Human bowel with a secondary perforation after laser irradiation.

Fig. 4. Wall compliance of the untreated (below) and the coagulated (above) bladder.

makes an essential contribution to the heating up of neighboring tissues. The two processes, thermal conduction and radiation scattering, cause the heated zone to spread both horizontally and in depth beyond the boundaries of the actual target zone. The influence of thermal conduction becomes evident with long irradiation times and that of scattering with high power densities.

In contrast to the bladder, the adjacent intestinal tissue exhibits greater absorption of the neodymium-YAG laser light and sensitiveness to temperature. Even temperatues of 60 °C, effective for about 2 s, cause damage associated with a dangerous risk of perforation [11]. The laser light has a depth of penetration of several millimeters, and approximately 10–20% of the radiation penetrates the normal wall. In consequence, even a laser power of only 55 W causes damage to adjacent intestinal loops, in the form of secondary perforation (fig. 3). In order to protect neighboring organs, the laser output power must be limited to 45 W in transurethral use.

For clinical application of the neodymium-YAG laser we investigated the visible change of tissue occurring during irradiation at the point of coagulation, i.e., the discoloration of the tissue surface. For this purpose we irradiated livers of rats in vivo both in air and under water, using a 5 mm wide parallel beam [10].

On applying a radiation energy of about 120 J in air, the depth of necrosis was 3 mm and independent of the time/power ratio. The surface turned white over an area corresponding to the cross section of the laser beam. Wider, but not deeper, necroses resulted when higher energies were used. Since we applied about 500 J, desiccation was followed by carbonization. Superficial white necroses (e.g., after electroresection) do not influence the in-depth shape of the laser necrosis configuration.

The results obtained with irradiation under water were completely different. Only from 500 J upward did discoloration of the surface become visible. The size of the discolored area is smaller than the diameter of the laser beam. Just below the surface a spherical coagulation necrosis isodiametric to the laser beam forms. By increasing the energy applied, the depth of the necrosis can be extended to more than 6 mm without carbonization of the surface. 'Paintbrush' irradiation produces overlapping and complete superficial and deep necroses. Bladder wall necrosis of about 30% is liable to occur with this procedure. After extensive irradiation of a minipig's bladder, we were unable to detect any changes in the passive compliance of the wall. Within the physiological range the hydrostatic capacity is not reduced. Beyond this range the capacity is reduced by about 30%. We observed wall perforation in the coagulated area only at pressures higher than 100 cm H_2O. Figure 4 shows the compliance of a normal and an irradiated bladder wall with linear behavior in the physiological range in each case. Perforation occurs earlier in the irradiated (upper) bladder in the nonelastic phase.

In an animal experiment we noted functionial changes in the bladder wall during the period of restitution after

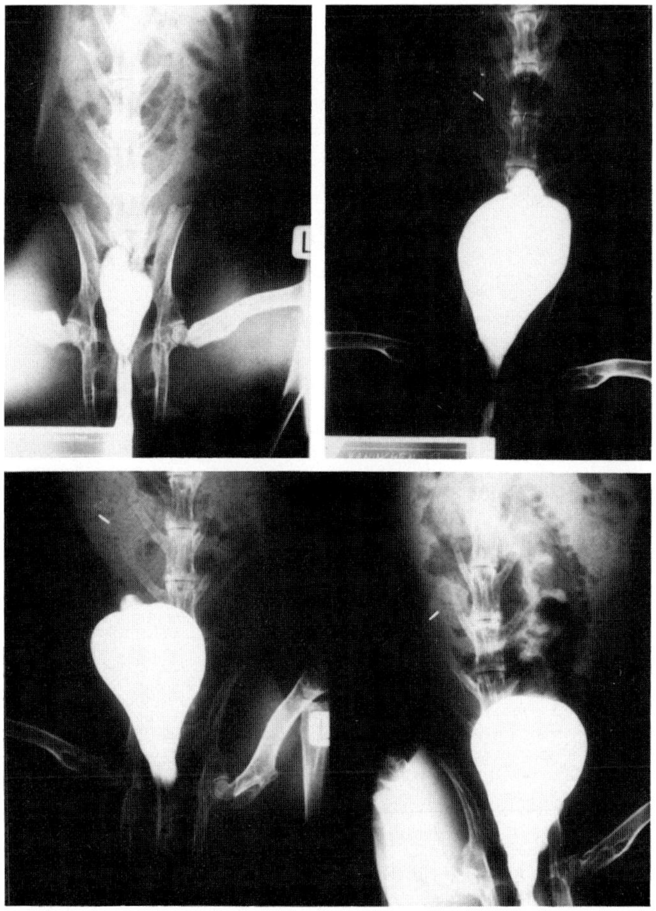

Fig. 5. Canine bladder 2 days (top, left), 4 days (top, right), 2 weeks (bottom, left), and 4 weeks (bottom, right) after laser coagulation.

extensive laser coagulation. Within the first 4 days the cystogram revealed large diverticula which had almost disappeared after 40 days (fig. 5). Table I summarizes the typical course of bladder restitution: 4 days after treatment diverticula formation is complete, with remarkable reduction in bladder volume and increase in compliance; after 40 days both volume and compliance are regular. There was no increase in detrusor activity. These findings correlate with the histologically monitored restitution of the bladder wall.

Summarizing, it may be stated that (1) the therapeutic effect of the neodymium-YAG laser is determined mainly by the product of laser output power and time of radiation; (2) to protect neighboring organs, the maximum laser output must be limited to 45 W; (3) the maximum depth of necroses is 3 mm in air and 6 mm under water, and (4) the therapeutic effect can be monitored on the basis of the superficial discoloration.

Table I. Changings of the bladder function after laser irradiation – Cystomanometry (animals)

Time	Volume	Compliance	Detrusor stability	Diverticulum
Preoperatively	normal	normal	+	∅
4 Days postoperatively	↓	↑	+	!
40 Days postoperatively	normal	normal	+	(+)

↓ = Reduced; ↑ = increased; + = yes; ∅ = no; (+) = only little.

References

1 Blazek, V.: Absorptions- und Streuverhalten biologischer Gewebe bezüglich der monochromatischen optischen Streuung. Adv. biomed. Technol. *24:* 331 (1979).

2 Bödecker, V.; Rudolph, M.; Groteluschen, B.: Messung der Intensitätsverteilung von YAG-Laserstrahlen im Gewebe. Adv. biomed. Technol. *19:* 160 (1974).

3 Eichler, J.; Knof, J.; Lenz, H.: Measurements on the depth of penetration of light (0.35–1.0 μm) in tissue. Radiat. environ. Biophys. *14:* 239 (1977).

4 Halldorsson, T.; Langerholc, J.: Thermodynamic analysis of laser irradiation of biological tissue, Appl. Optics *17:* 3948 (1978).

5 Hofstetter, A.G.; Frank, F.: The neodymium-YAG laser in urology (Hoffmann-La Roche, Basel 1980).

6 Hu, C.; Barnes, F.S.: The thermal-chemical damage in biological material under laser irradiation. JEEE-BME *17:* 220 (1970).

7 Keiditsch, E.: Histologische Grundlagen der endoskopischen Neodym-YAG-Laserbestrahlung. Urologe A *20:* 300 (1981).

8 McCord, R.C.; Weinberg, W.; Gorisch, W.; Leheta, F.; Schönberger, J.L.: Thermal effets in laser irradiated biological tissue. Proc. Symp. Laser, in Medicine and Biology, Neuherberg 1977).

9 Pensel, J.; Hofstetter, A.G.; Frank, F.; Keiditsch, E.; Rothenberger, K.: Temporal and spatial temperature profile of the bladder serose in intravesical neodymium-YAG laser irradiation. Eur. Urol. *7:* 298 (1981).

10 Rothenberger, K.; Pensel, J.; Hofstetter, A.G.; Keiditsch, E.; Stern, J.: Dosierung der Neodym-YAG-Laserbestrahlung zur endovesikalen Anwendung bei Blasentumoren. Urologe A *20:* 310 (1981).

11 Staehler, G.; Halldorrson, T.; Langerholc, J.; Bilgram, R.: Dosimetry for neodymium-YAG laser applications in urology. Lisam *1:* 191 (1980).

J. Pensel,
Department of Urology,
Medical University of Lübeck,
Ratzeburger Allee 160,
D-2400 Lübeck 1 (FRG)

Eur. Urol. *12:* suppl. 1, pp. 21–24 (1986)

0302–2838/86/0127–0021$2.75/0

Treatment of Urological Tumors by Neodymium-YAG Laser

A. Hofstetter

Urological Department, Medical University of Lübeck, FRG

Key Words. Urological tumors · Neodymium-YAG laser · Condylomata acuminata · Adjuvant chemotherapy · Penile cancer

Abstract. Our 9-year clinical experience with the neodymium-YAG laser permits us to state that the conventional methods of tumor treatment in urology should be reconsidered for urothelial tumors. In benign tumors of the genitals and penile cancer the laser application is superior to all other conventional methods of treatment.

Introduction

On the basis of our 13 years of experience with lasers, including numerous experiments and attempts to utilize lasers in urology, the only application that has endured is the destruction of benign and malignant tumors of the external genitals and tumors of the urethral, vesical, and ureteral mucosa by the neodymium-YAG (Nd:YAG) laser used through the endoscope or in open surgery. Cancers of the renal pelvis can also be destroyed by the Nd:YAG laser.

Apart fom the Nd:YAG laser, laser photoradiation is also of interest in the diagnosis and treatment of bladder cancer [1, 3].

Techniques

Endoscopic destruction of bladder tumors is carried out in three steps if the tumors are bulky. In these cases, the exophytic portion is first resected with the electric snare deep into the bladder wall after prior coagulation of the margins of the tumor. The base and edges of the tumor are then postcoagulated with the Nd:YAG laser.

Smaller tumors are primarily destroyed with the Nd:YAG laser. Here, we first irradiate until blanching of the tissue surrounding the tumor occurs to a breadth of about 0.5–1 cm, in order to seal off the afferent blood vessels and lymphatics. Subsequently, the tumor is necrotized linearly.

Immediately after irradiation, the tumor is removed with biopsy forceps. This tissue removed immediately after the Nd:YAG irradiation can be subject to histological workup to confirm the diagnosis and to classify the tumor.

Before the operation, biopsies are taken from the base of the tumor and the tissue immediately surrounding the tumor for a distance of 1 cm at 3, 6, 9, and 12 o'clock. This procedure is supplemented by 'quadrant biopsy'.

Since no, or only very insignificant, hemorrhage occurs under Nd:YAG laser irradiation, a transurethral catheter can as a rule be dispensed with after the operation. This is important in avoiding nosocomial infections.

The patient should be kept under observation for 1 day after the operation, in order to detect a possible intestinal perforation in good time, in particular when large areas are irradiated at the posterior wall of the bladder. With a radiation dose of up to 45 W, using water as a flushing fluid, we have yet to observe such a complication, although we have treated several thousands tumors. Within 8 years only in 3 cases did small intestinal perforations occur after faulty irradiation at too high a power (about 80 W). Clinically, these perforations manifested as signs of acute abdomen within 12 h after the irradiation.

Table I. Primary tumors (pT_A–pT_2, N_0, M_0)

n	Sex		Age, years			
	males	females	males		females	
			range	mean	range	mean
40	23	17	45–81	66.5	54–81	69.1

Table II. Relapse tumors (pT_A–pT_2, N_0, M_0)

n	Sex		Age, years			
	males	females	males		females	
			range	mean	range	mean
26	16	10	40–79	62.1	53–83	72.1

Table III. Classification and incidence distribution of transitional cell carcinomas in 20 (M = 12/F = 8) patients of the laser group and 20 (M = 11/F = 9) patients of the TUR group

	Laser group				TUR group			
pT/G	1	2	3	n	1	2	3	n
A	7	3	0	10	7	5	0	12
1	4	3	1	8	1	0	3	4
2	0	0	2	2	1	2	1	4

Table IV. Classification and incidence distribution of transitional cell carcinoma in 20 (M = 12/F = 8) patients of the laser group and 6 (M = 4/F = 2) patients of the TUR group

	Laser group				TUR group			
pT/G	1	2	3	n	1	2	3	n
A	3	3	0	6	1	3	0	4
1	5	6	3	14	1	1	0	2
2	0	0	0	0	0	0	0	0

Clinical Results

Since 1976, we have treated more than 600 patients with stage pT_A, $pT_{1/2}$, and pT_3 bladder tumors with the Nd:YAG laser. The local relapse rate varied between 1 and 5% in contrast to transurethral resection (TUR) with a recidivation rate of 40–60% in the world literature [5–7]. The advantage of this technique is contact-free tumor destruction under excellent visual conditions, since there is no or only slight hemorrhage during the operation.

The operation does not require general anesthesia. In most cases appropriate sedation suffices so that the operation can also be carried out on an outpatient basis.

The (sometimes very expensive) electrolyte-free flushing solutions can be replaced by sterile water, thus saving costs.

Apart from these advantages, the question as to the efficacy of the Nd:YAG laser as compared with conventional TUR techniques also needed to be investigated. In a prospective randomized study, we have compared the efficacy of the laser with the results obtained with TUR – using the rate of recurrence as a criterion. Patients with stage pT_A–pT_2, N_0, M_0 urothelial carcinomas (n = 66; 39 men, 27 women; average age 68 years) were included in the study. Laser or TUR treatment was carried out in accordance with a randomization scheme.

In addition, adjuvant chemotherapy with mitomycin C (20 mg/14 days) was administered 8 days after the operation. The control group received no chemoprophylaxis. The study was commenced on September 1, 1981. The patients were divided into a group with primary tumors (table I) and a group with relapse tumors (table II). The classification of primary tumors is shown in table III and the classification of relapse tumors in table IV.

The therapeutic results obtained in primary tumors are shown in table V. It can be seen that laser application with and without chemotherapy is superior to TUR with and without chemotherapy, as indicated by the relapse rate ($p < 0.0001$). The superiority of laser application was also seen in relapse tumors (table VI). In addition, a particularly important observation is, we believe, that after laser application hardly any local relapses occurred in contrast to TUR (~1 to ~40%). Otherwise it is interesting to note that there was never any change from localized to multiple tumor growth after laser irradiation, unlike TUR. Our experience has been confirmed in general by Meier et al. [4].

Other Urothelial Tumors

Besides the destruction of urothelial carcinomas of the urinary bladder, we were also able to destroy tumors in the ureter in patients in whom a more radical surgical

Table V. Therapeutic results after Nd:YAG laser coagulation versus TUR (n = 40)

	Laser + mitomycin (n = 15)	Laser alone (n = 9)	TUR + mitomycin (n = 13)	TUR alone (n = 3)
Number of patients with recurrence	1	1	6	3
Recurrence rate[a]	0.27	0.41	2.44	10.71
Mean follow-up time, months	24.97	27.11	18.92	9.33
Deaths	1[b]	0	1[b]	0
Total follow-up time, months	374.5	244.0	246.0	28.0

[a] $\text{Recurrence rate} = \frac{\text{number of recurrences}}{\text{months follow-up}} \times 100.$

[b] Not due to cancer.

Table VI. Therapeutic results after Nd:YAG laser coagulation versus TUR (n = 26)

	Laser + mitomycin (n = 15)	Laser alone (n = 5)	TUR + mitomycin (n = 2)	TUR alone (n = 4)
Number of patients with recurrence	2	5	2	3
Recurrence rate[a]	0.75	2.44	7.14	11.1
Mean follow-up time, months	20.4	23.4	14.0	9.0
Deaths	0	0	0	0
Total follow-up time, months	306	117	28	36

[a] $\text{Recurrence rate} = \frac{\text{number of recurrences}}{\text{months follow-up}} \times 100.$

Table VII. Clinical results after coagulation of ureteral tumors (N_0, M_0) with the Nd:YAG laser

Patient No.	Age years	Sex	Diagnosis (G/St)	Laser coagulation I	Observation period, months	Relapse after months	Further steps
001	62	male	m. BTp + UT, r (G_1/pT_1; O → U = 4 cm)	5,819	39	no	–
002	58	male	m. BT_R + UT_{b+r} (G_2/pT_1; O → U = 3 cm)	8,225	40	no	–
003	65	male	$UT_{(stump)}$ (G_1/pT_A; O → U = 3 cm)	4,131	40	no	–
004	71	male	m. BT_p + UT_r (G_1, pT_1; O → U = 4 cm)	5,903	38	no	–
005	82	female	UT, 1 (G_2/pT_2; O → U = 3 cm)	4,712	27	yes (after 14 months)	laser coagulation

BT = Bladder tumor; p = primary; UT = Ureter tumor; O = ostium; U = ureter; R = relapse.

procedure was not indicated. Thus, we treated 5 patients with ureter tumors (G_1–G_2, pT_1–pT_2).

All our patients are still alive. There was only 1 relapse, so that recoagulation with Nd:YAG laser became necessary. The patient has been free of recurrent disease for more than 14 months (table VII). Furthermore, 2 patients with kidney pelvis tumors were also treated by Nd:YAG laser (table VIII).

Our experience with laser coagulation of ureter and renal pelvis tumors is small, but our observation period is more than 3 years, and our results have been good, especially in the case of ureter tumors.

This organ-preserving method appears suitable for noninvasive tumors of all types of malignancy without metastases. A problem in some cases might be the endoscopic handling and the possibility of missing tumor

Table VIII. Clinical results after coagulation of renal pelvis tumors ($N_{x/0}$, M_0) with the Nd:YAG laser

Patient No.	Age years	Sex	Diagnosis (G/St)	Laser coagulation I	Observation period, months	Relapse after months	Further steps
100	72	male	RPT, r (Rest K; G_2/pT_2)	4,312 (PCF)	35	6	laser coagulation
101	80	female	RPT, l (G_2/pT_2)	5,314 (OS)	3	–	–

RPT = Relapse, primary tumor; PCF = percutaneous fistula; OS = open surgery.

areas. Therefore, these tumor patients must be monitored very closely. This is possible with the new ureteroscopic techniques. The main indications for this procedure are high-risk patients with superficial small tumor areas in the ureter or with small tumors in renal pelvis or calyx. Further, bleeding tumors or inflammatory bleeding areas.

The success rate in laser treatment of urethral and genital condylomata acuminata in 493 cases was 97%. 93% had been pretreated with other therapeutic methods, but without success.

Of our 17 patients with penile cancer (pT_1–pT_2, N_0, M_0) only 1 died of metastatic disease. He was obviously understaged at time of treatment. The observation period extends from 2.5 to 5.5 years.

References

1 Benson, R.: Use of HpD in the treatment of neoplastic diseases (this symposium).

2 Hofstetter, A.; Frank, F.; Keiditsch, E.; Wondrazek, F.: Intracorporale, laserinduzierte Stosswellen-Lithotripsie (ILISL). Laser *1:* 155–158 (1985).

3 Jocham, D.; Schmiedt, E.; Staehler, G.: Laser-photodynamic therapy of multifocal bladder carcinoma using hematoporphyrin derivative (HpD) as a tumor photosensitizer. XXth Congr. Int. Soc. Urol., Vienna 1985.

4 Meier, U.; Hofstetter, A.; Pflüger, H.: Effects of intravesical instillation of mitomycin after endoscopic treatment with TUR or laser on recurrence rate of bladder tumors. XXth Congr. Int. Soc. Urol., Vienna 1985.

5 Page, B.H.; Levison, U.B.; Corwen, M.P.: The site of recurrence of non-infiltrating bladder tumors. Br. J. Urol. *50:* 237 (1978).

6 Weldon, T.E.; Soloway, M.S.: Susceptibility of urothelium to neoplastic cellular implantation. Urology *5:* 824 (1975).

7 Zingg, E.J.: Maligne Tumoren der Harnblase; in Hohenfellner, Zingg, Urologie, vol. I (Thieme, Stuttgart 1982).

Prof. A. Hofstetter,
Urologische Klinik und Poliklinik der
Medizinischen Universität zu Lübeck,
Ratzeburger Allee 160,
D–2400 Lübeck 1 (FRG)

Eur. Urol. 12: suppl. 1, pp. 25–27 (1986)

0302–2838/86/0127–0025$2.75/0

Neodymium-YAG Laser in Transitional Cell Cancer of the Bladder with Emphasis on Outpatient Potential

Terrence R. Malloy

Section of Urology, Pennsylvania Hospital, Philadelphia, Pa., USA

Key Words. Neodymium-YAG laser · Ancillary treatment · Chemotherapy · Radiations

Abstract. With ever-increasing medical costs in the United States, the neodymium-YAG laser has afforded urologists the opportunity to treat the vast majority of patients with superficial transitional cell carcinoma of the bladder (T0, T1, T2) as outpatients. This has significantly decreased medical costs as well as patient loss of income. Seventy-six patients with superficial transitional cell carcinoma of the bladder were treated solely with the neodymium-YAG laser and followed for at least 2 years. No patient received ancillary treatment, chemotherapy, or radiation. Forty-eight patients (63%) had no evidence of recurrent tumors when followed for 2 years or longer. Twenty-eight patients (37%) had recurrent tumors. Only 3 patients (4%) had an increase in stage. There were no major complications in this group of patients. Seventy percent of the patients were treated as outpatients or 1-day hospital admissions.

Superficial transitional cell carcinoma of the bladder (T0, T1, T2) has been traditionally treated in the United States of America with electrocautery transurethral resection of the bladder tumors. This type of treatment has required a hospital stay averaging between 3 and 5 days. Five-year survival rates in this group of patients have varied between 62 and 80% [1]. But recurrence rates have been extremely high, ranging from 48 to 70% [2]. Complications with the electrocautery resection of bladder tumors have included bleeding, bladder perforation, long use of catheters and urinary tract infections. With ever-increasing medical costs in the United States, the neodymium-YAG laser presented a method of treating superficial transitional cell cancers of the bladder with fewer chances of complication and the possibility of treating the patients as outpatients or 1-day admissions. In 1981 Hofstetter [3] reported on 302 bladder tumors treated with the neodymium-YAG laser. With a recurrence rate of less than 10%, and minimal operative complications, this form of therapy appeared to have unique qualities suitable for eradication of transitional cell carcinoma of the bladder. In an effort to evaluate the effectiveness of the neodymium-YAG laser in treating patients with superficial transitional cell carcinoma of the bladder (T0, T1, T2) 76 patients were treated and followed for at least 2 years. The majority of patients were treated as outpatients or 1-day hospital admissions.

Material and Methods

Seventy-six patients with superficial transitional cell carcinoma of the bladder were treated with tumoricidal doses of photoradiation from the neodymium-YAG laser. Forty males and 16 females had T0 and T1 lesions, while 12 males and 8 females had T2 carcinomas of the bladder. All patients were staged identically with the following studies: (1) intravenous pyelography, (2) complete bimanual pelvic examination; (3) cystoscopy with biopsy; (4) ultrasound and/or abdominal pelvic computerized axial tomography scans in any patients where staging was questionable, and (5) urine cytology.

After biopsies were obtained and staging completed, all lesions were treated endoscopically with the neodymium-YAG laser light source through a cystoscope or resectoscope. In tumors larger than

2.5 cm, transurethral resection of the major part of the mass was accomplished and then followed by neodymium-YAG laser photoradiation in tumoricidal doses. Lesions less than 2.5 cm in diameter were biopsied with 'cold punch' biopsy forceps and then treated with the laser.

The power settings used for the tumoricidal therapy were within the range recommended by Hofstetter [3], Keiditsch et al. [4], and Rothenberger et al. [5] which had been established through studies on animal, cadaver, and cystectomy bladder specimens. All carcinomas were treated within a power range of 35–40 W with time intervals not exceeding 3 s on anyone area of the tumor. Care was taken to prevent forward scatter of the thermal energy to small-bowel contents adjacent to the bladder which might have caused bowel perforations. The individual lesions were treated initially in a circumferential fashion around the base. When all the lymphatics were sealed, the lesion was treated until it became pale white in color, corresponding to the state of protein denaturation within the tumor. The tumors sloughed from the bladder over the following 6–14 days.

Seventy percent of the patients were treated as outpatients or 1-day hospital admissions. Those that required anesthesia had their procedure early in the morning and remained in an outpatient area until it was determined that they had voided and were having no abdominal pain. They would then be discharged. Thirty percent were treated as 2-day or longer inpatient hospitalizations.

All patients had urine cytology and follow-up cystoscopies at 3-month intervals for at least 2 years. None of the patients received chemotherapy, radiation, or any other form of supplemental therapy.

Results

All patients were followed for at least 2 years or longer after the initial neodymium-YAG laser photoradiation therapy. Forty-eight patients (63%) had no evidence of recurrent tumors or positive cytologies when followed for more than 2 years. Twenty-eight patients (37%) had recurrent cancers. Three patients (4%) had an increase of stage: 1 patient T0 increased to T1, while 2 patients with T1 increased to T2. Six patients had recurrent tumors in the 3- to 6-month postoperative period. Six patients (8%) had recurrences within the 6- to 12-month period. Fourteen patients (18%) had recurrences between 12 and 24 months. Thirty-eight patients with T0, T1 superficial tumor (68%) had no evidence of recurrence within the 24-month period. Ten patients (50%) with T2 lesions had no evidence of recurrences within the first 2 years.

There were no major complications in this group of patients. There were no bladder perforations and no instances of bowel perforation. Two patients experienced ileus which resolved within 36 h. There were no episodes of urinary sepsis. Postoperatively the patients' hemoglobin levels remained stable. None of the patients treated on an outpatient basis required subsequent readmission to the hospital for complications.

Discussion

Transurethral resection of bladder tumors with electrocautery has led to high recurrence rates because of several factors suggested by Hinman [6]: (1) seeding of viable transitional cell carcinomas into the raw mucosal areas of the bladder from the resection or areas of the bladder traumatized by instrumentation; (2) increased vulnerability of resected areas to carcinogens or resected tumor cells, (3) failure to resect all visible tumors; (4) tumors present but not visible, and (5) continued activity of the carcinogens in the urine.

Failure to resect all visible tumors should be eliminated by experienced surgeons. Tumors present but not visible and continued activity of the carcinogen in the urine are difficult problems to eliminate. However, seeding of transitional cell carcinomas by electrocautery resection and trauma has to be a major concern as shown by several series [7–9].

The neodymium-YAG laser has unique qualities which makes it advantageous in the treatment of superficial transitional cell carcinoma of the bladder in the outpatient or short-procedure unit: (1) the neodymium-YAG laser photoradiation can be delivered by fiberoptic light guides through standard urologic endoscopes and does not require special intrumentation; (2) the neodymium-YAG laser is not impeded by water or urine; (3) the neodymium-YAG-laser produces deep uniform scatter throughout the bladder muscle producing hemogeneous and uniform distribution of photoradiation to the carcinoma inducing a thermal effect deep into the underlying bladder muscle; (4) contactless and bloodless destruction of the superficial transitional cell carcinoma permits outpatient or short-procedure therapy; (5) the absence of electric power flowing through the tissue avoids muscle contraction of the bladder and potential obturator nerve reflex spasms; (6) when used at the proper power settings, there is no chance of bladder perforation with neodymium-YAG laser photoradiation; (7) there is no trauma to normal mucosa of the bladder or prostatic urethra in males; (8) catheters are not required postoperatively, thus decreasing the potential for urinary tract infection; (9) patients can be treated under local anesthesia, or, if required, general anesthesia can be used in the outpatient operating suite – the subsequent savings to the medical insurance carriers are substantial, and (10) patient rehabilitation is prompt, as most patients are able to return to work immediately.

In this group of 76 patients followed for at least 2 years the overall recurrence rate has been 37%. In long-term analysis, the recurrence rate of tumors in patients treated with the neodymium-YAG laser may not differ appreciably from those that are treated with electrocautery resection. However, the neodymium-YAG laser certainly has proven itself as effective as electrocautery resection for superficial transitional cell carcinoma of the bladder. Lack of complications, the ability to be used in the outpatient setting, and decreased costs make it an attractive alternative in the treatment of superficial cancer of the bladder. Long-term assessment in multiple institutions is necessary to evaluate the true efficacy of the neodymium-YAG laser in treating cancer of the bladder. With 70% of patients treated as outpatients or 1-day hospital stay patients, the costs to the third-party insurance carriers or government agencies have been significantly reduced.

References

1 Prout, G.R.: Superficial bladder cancer, in Smith, Prout, Bladder cancer, chapter 9, pp. 151–171 (Butterworth, London 1984).

2 Soloway, M.S.: The management of superficial bladder cancer. Cancer *45:* 1856 (1980).

3 Hofstetter, A.: Endoskopische Zerstörungen von Blasentumoren mit Laser. Urologe A *20:* 317 (1981).

4 Keiditsch, F.; Hofstetter, A.; Zimmerman, I.; Stern, J.; Frank, F.; Babaryka, I.: Histological investigation to substantiate the therapy of bladder tumors with the neodymium-YAG Laser. Laser *1:* 19 (1985).

5 Rothenberger, K.; Pensel, J.; Hofstetter, A.; et al.: Transurethral laser coagulation for treatment of urinary bladder tumors. Laser Surg. Med. *2:* 255 (1983).

6 Hinman, F., Jr.: The recurrence of bladder tumors. J. Urol. *83:* 294 (1960).

7 Weldon, T.E.; Soloway, M.S.; Persky, L.: Urothelial susceptibility to neoplastic cellular implantation. Surg. Forum *25:* 547 (1974).

8 Page, B.H.; Levision, V.B.; Curwen, M.P.: The site of recurrence of non-infiltrating tumors. Br. J. Urol. *50:* 237 (1978).

9 Boyd, P.J.R.; Burnand, K.G.: Site of bladder tumor recurrence. Lancet *ii:* 1290 (1974).

T.R. Malloy, MD,
Section of Urology,
Pennsylvania Hospital,
299 S 8th Street,
Philadelphia, PA 19106 (USA)

Eur. Urol. *12:* suppl. 1, pp. 28–29 (1986)

Percutaneous Laser Therapy of Tumors of the Upper Urinary Tract

G. Hutschenreiter

Urologische Klinik der Evangelischen und Johanniter-Krankenanstalten Duisburg-Nord, Oberhausen, BRD

Key Words. Bilateral tumor involvement · Palliative therapy · Percutaneous laser irradiation

Abstract. The small number of patients I have treated to date permit only a preliminary report on the results obtained. So far, 3 patients with a mean age of 68 years have been treated, including 1 case of bilateral tumor involvement. One female patient was irradiated three times. Here, therapy was primarily of palliative nature. At least as a form of palliative therapy, percutaneous laser irradiation appears to be a valuable alternative in apparently hopeless cases. Since we may assume that we are still far removed from what is technically feasible, we should also investigate percutaneous laser therapy with regard to its curative effects.

Compared with those for carcinoma of the renal pelvis, the possibilities for the treatment of urinary bladder carcinoma are manifold. This is undoubtedly due to the anatomic conditions involved.

Over the past few years technical developments have opened up new possibilities that permit us to reconsider our concept of therapy for urothelial tumors of the kidney.

Extensive experience with percutaneous renal stone operations has made endoscopic access to the renal collecting system so reliable that a similar differentiated therapeutic approach may be used in the kidneys as in the bladder. If the tumor cannot be accessed via the ureter by means of ureterorenoscopy, a percutaneous nephrostomy channel is established. As in the bladder, cold or hot biopsy is used for staging and grading.

The main differences between bladder and kidney are the close proximity of major vessels in the kidneys and the relatively thin muscular layer of the pyelocaliceal system as compared with the bladder.

Although percutaneous electroresection of tumors of the renal pelvis is necessary to reduce the mass of large exophytic tumors, it also carries with it the danger of major vessel injury and massive bleeding when applied to the tumor bed. To this must be added the already constrained space of the renal cavity. The contactless use of the neodymium-YAG laser in the kidney, therefore, represents a real alternative, the advantages of which are not as readily evident in the bladder. Contactless laser irradiation also ensures good visibility of the operating field. Unlike the laser, high-frequency current alone does not have a suffciently deep necrotizing effect. However, as is well known, the factor imposing limitations on the laser is the size of the tumor. Within the past 18 months percutaneous laser therapy has been carried out in 3 patients with urothelial tumors.

Case Reports

In a 77-year-old female patient three irradiation series were conducted with 19,000, 40,000, and 16,000 J at an output power of about 40 W. The patient had a conservatively preoperated solitary kidney. Owing to the patient's advanced age, her refusal to undergo nephrectomy, and the fact that only 1 kidney was functional, it was

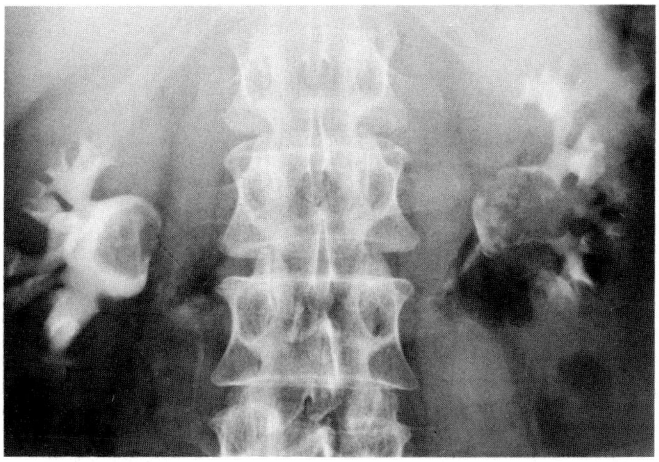

Fig. 1. 68-year-old man with bilateral renal pelvic tumors (pT_A grade I).

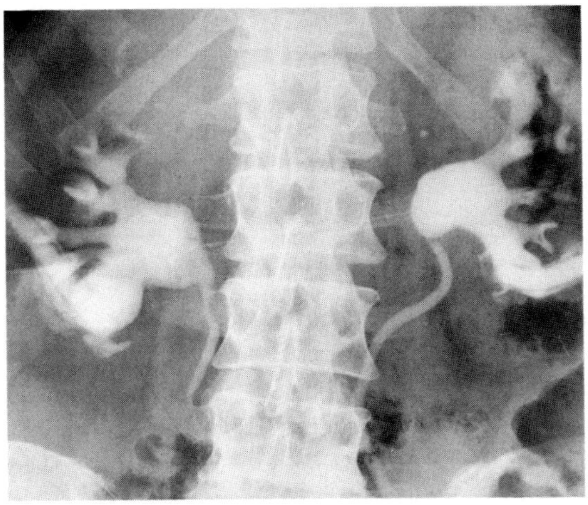

Fig. 2. 68-year-old man with bilateral renal pelvic tumors. Condition after percutaneous electroresection and bilateral laser irradiation.

necessary to institute organ-preserving therapy with palliative intent. A partial resection had been carried out 3 years previously to remove a T_A grade I tumor.

Because of recurrent tumors in the bladder and distal ureter, transurethral resections have since been carried out in the bladder, as well as resection of the distal ureter. A ring nephrostomy keeps open the endoscopic channel to the kidney for urine drainage and for any subsequent endoscopic laser therapy. Urea and creatinine levels in the patient did not rise as a result of the laser therapy. Nor was any appreciable bleeding observed.

In a 50-year-old patient, a small T_A grade I tumor of the right kidney was irradiated percutanously with curative intent. In view of the patient's relative youthfulness and the presence of a healthy contralateral kidney, a nephrectomy was performed when a pea-size recurrent tumor appeared 3 months later.

In a 68-year-old male patient with bilateral tumor involvement (T_A grade I; fig. 1), the exophytic tumor masses were electroresected on both sides. The tumor bed was then irradiated at a power output of 40 W with 7,000 J on the right side and 10,000 J on the left. The patient was discharged with bilateral nephrostomies (fig. 2).

An endoscopic follow-up examination including bilateral biopsies done 8 weeks later showed no evidence of tumor recurrence. The nephrostomy channels were removed. Monthly urinary cytologic tests and quarterly endoscopic checks (ureterorenoscopy) are planned for follow-up.

Prof. G. Hutschenreiter,
Urologische Abteilung,
Akademisches Lehrkrankenhaus der Universität Düsseldorf,
Steinbrinkstrasse 96a,
D-4200 Oberhausen 11 (FRG)

Eur. Urol. *12:* suppl. 1, pp. 30–33 (1986)

0302–2838/86/0127–0030$2.75/0

Use of the Neodymium-YAG Laser in the Treatment of Ureteral Tumors and Urethral Condylomata acuminata

Clinical Experience

A. Schilling[a], *R. Böwering*[a], *E. Keiditsch*[b]

[a] Department of Urology (Director: Priv. Doz. Dr. A. Schilling), and
[b] Pathologic Institute (Director: Dr. E. Keiditsch), Municipal Hospital, Munich-Bogenhausen, Munich, FRG

Key Words. Laser coagulation · Ureteral carcinoma · Urethral condylomata acuminata · Strictures

Abstract. The further development of endoscopic instruments has made neodymium-YAG laser irradiation of ureteral tumors possible. To date a total of 13 ureteral tumors in 10 patients have been photocoagulated. Over a mean follow-up period of 23 months, only 1 heterotopic recurrence was found after 14 months. In view of the results achieved so far, nephroureterectomy as the first therapeutic step appears to have been made obsolete. Since 1979 we have treated 48 patients with the neodymium-YAG laser. Seven patients with excessive condyloma involvement were followed postoperatively. Our experience indicates that, in view of its low complication and recurrence rates, endoscopic laser coagulation of urethral condylomata is the method of choice. A short-term ureteroscopic follow-up examination, however, is required to detect any condylomata that might have been overlooked.

Introduction

The further development of endoscopic instruments and the possibility of coupling these to flexible quartz-glass light guides makes the entire urinary tract accessible to laser therapy. Today it is possible to operate within the entire urinary tract system under virtually identical conditions as in the bladder. With this in mind, we decided to use the neodymium-YAG laser to perform organ-preserving coagulation of ureteral tumors.

Involvement of the urethra with condylomata acuminata constitutes a most difficult therapeutic problem for which a satisfactory solution has proved elusive. The long-term results of current conservative therapeutic measures and surgical techniques are associated with a high recurrence rate. In addition, there is a high risk of the caustic agents used being absorbed or of finding their way into other areas, perhaps leading to fatal incidents [2, 8, 9, 13, 16]. The classical operative measures result in considerable damage to the urethra, ranging from high-grade strictures to fistulas. In extreme cases the entire urethra has had to be split. After laser coagulation was applied with considerable success to the treatment of external condylomata, we felt justified in using the technique in the treatment of condylomata acuminata of the urethra [3, 6, 7, 12].

Laser coagulation of ureteral tumors and condylomata acuminata of the urethra presents common problems. For example, only tangential impingement of the laser beam is possible in both cases. Furthermore, strictures must be feared as a complication of operations on tubular organs, especially when thermal measures are used. The following is a report of our initial experience.

Materials and Methods

Ureteral Tumors

The diagnosis was based on infusion urograms, retrograde imaging of the affected ureter and abdominal or pelvic computed tomography for tumor staging. Histologic examination was performed with a Storz ureteroscope after a guide wire had been advanced past the ureteral tumor into the renal pelvis. Using this wire running through the working channel as a guide, the telescope was advanced up to a point just distal to the ureteral tumor. Any obstructions were dilated with Teflon bougies, again using the same guide wire. As soon as the ureteroscope was focused on the tumor, the guide wire was replaced with flexible biopsy forceps to obtain tissue specimens.

In this manner classification of all the tumors was accomplished, including infiltration depths and histologic grade. Immediately after biopsy, laser coagulation of the tumor was performed through the same ureteroscope. This instrument, modified in accordance with Perez-Castro and Martinez-Pineiro [11], has a sheath diameter of 11

French, and an overall length of 390 mm. The laser light guide is passed down the irrigation channel next to the antegrade telescope. The quartz-glass fiber guide is mobile and can be advanced or withdrawn as required. To prevent kinking of the thin ureteroscope sheath with resulting impairment of the visual field, we had a 17-French guide sheath developed. With the help of this sheath, bladder filling can also be easily regulated. The tumor was irradiated with a neodymium-YAG laser at a distance of 1–2 mm, under low-pressure irrigation. A power output of 40 W with a pulse duration of 1–3 s was used. Blanching and shrinkage of the tumor (already known in bladder tumors) were interpreted as signs that coagulation necrosis had occurred. The coagulated tumor can usually be removed with the blunt end of the instrument, so that the smooth tumor base and the surrounding area are exposed for further laser coagulation. Then, irradiation of the so-called shadow areas, which are accessible only after removal of the tumor, can be effected [1]. Irradiation of the surrounding tissue is intended to prevent tumor cell dissemination.

Since November 1981, 12 patients (7 male, 5 female) with a total of 16 ureteral tumors were treated with the above-described technique. The mean age of the patients was 67.3 years. In the first series the method was restricted to patients who refused conventional surgery, or in whom surgery was contraindicated by the presence of disease. Since January 1985, however, we have been treating all ureteral tumors with this technique. All the tumors were located in the lower ureter and were nonmetastatic with a low malignancy grade (GI–GII) and at an infiltration stage that did not exceed pT_1. Eight tumors were located on the right, 8 on the left. One patient had bilateral tumors, 2 other patients had tumors in both sections of a ureteral fissure, and 1 patient had two isolated unilateral tumors. In 5 cases an indwelling splint was inserted immediately after laser exposure due to the extent of the coagulation area.

Condylomata acuminata

Since 1979, 48 patients with more or less pronounced condylomatous involvement of the urethra were treated endoscopically at our clinic with the neodymium-YAG laser. The irradiation energy was determined primarily by the endoscopic clinical picture. The appearance of a white necrosis served as the criterion of successful coagulation. The mean coagulation energy applied was 40 W, with a pulse duration of approximately 2 s.

To assessing the clinical value of the technique, we selected only 7 patients from the series, all of whom had extensive involvement of the entire urethra (bulbar urethra to the external meatus; fig. 1). In 1 case the external sphincter and the prostatic urethra were also affected with condylomata. The mean age of the patients was 32 years (21–67 years).

To clear the urethra completely of tumors, 3–4 sessions were required. The follow-up examinations were performed first at 3-month and later at 6-month intervals.

1

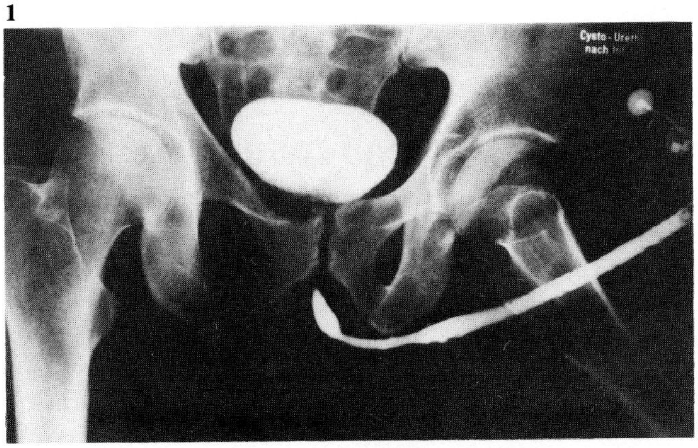

2a 2b

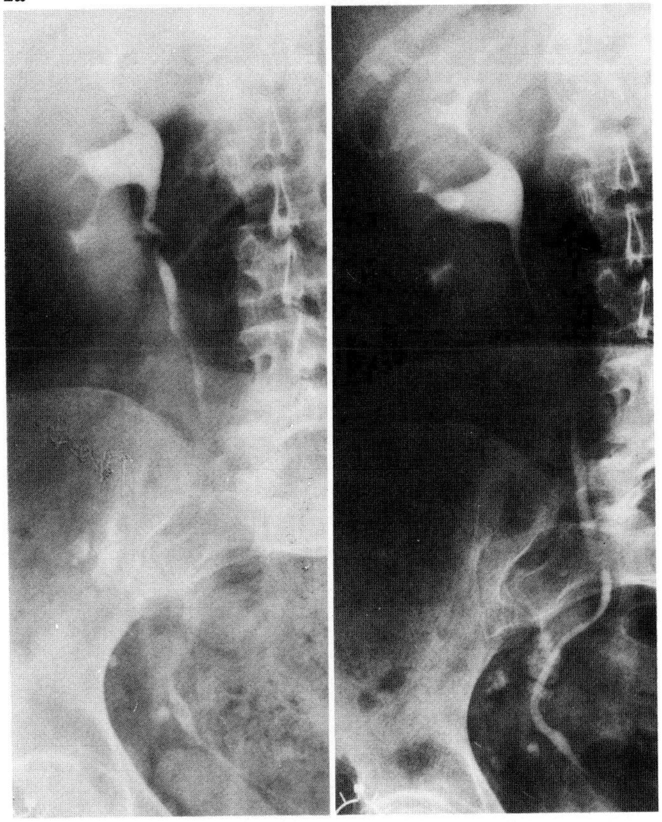

Fig. 1. Extensive involvement of the entire urethra with condylomata acuminata in a 40-year-old man.

Fig. 2. An 81-year-old woman with a pea-sized ureteral tumor: before (**a**) and after (**b**) endoscopic laser coagulation.

Results

Ureteral Tumors

Laser irradiation of the ureteral tumors was extremely well tolerated by all patients. In no case did fever episodes occur. Happily, no injuries of the neighboring organs were found. Preoperative tumor-related drainage obstructions were no longer detected in any urogram taken 6 weeks postoperatively. Also, no radiation-induced stenosis of the ureter occurred – even after removal of the indwelling splints (fig. 2a, b).

Epithelialization of the defect, as was documented in a ureterectomy specimen (nephroureterocystectomy for an invasive GIII tumor), was complete just 3 weeks after

3 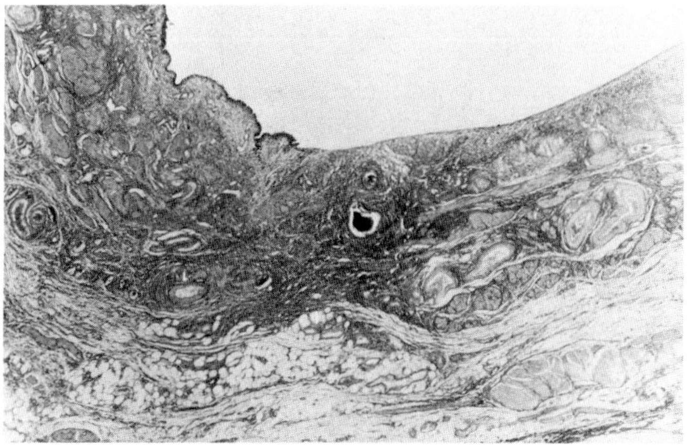

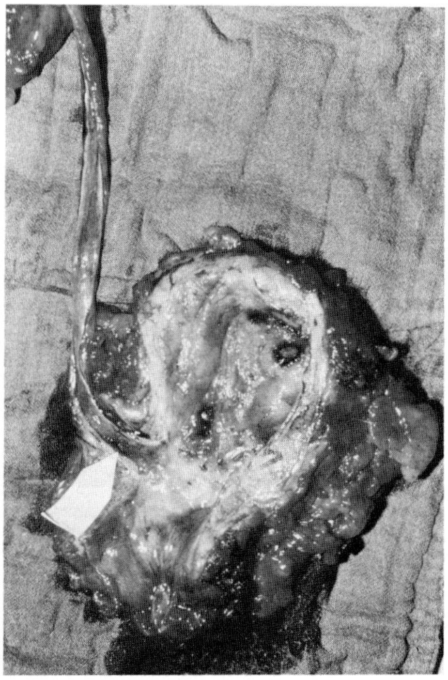 4

Fig. 3. Epithelialization of the ureter 3 weeks after laser coagulation. No tumor cells are now evident.

Fig. 4. Nephroureterocystoprostatectomy biopsy. Condition following recurrent invasive bladder tumors. Condition 3 weeks after laser coagulation of a ureteral tumor (GIII; white arrow). No evidence of stenosis, perforation or injury of neighboring structures.

laser coagulation (fig. 3). The absence of the above-mentioned potential complications was documented by means of intraoperative biopsies (fig. 4).

Over a mean follow-up period of 23 months (3–31 months), no local tumor recurrences were observed. Only in 1 patient was a recurrence found after 14 months, a cherry-sized bladder tumor directly on the right ostium which had spread approximately 2 cm intramurally. The site of the original laser-coagulated tumor was proximal to this.

Condylomata acuminata

The mean follow-up period is 1.9 years (6 months to 5 years). At present 4 patients are free of condylomata after an average of three laser sessions. Two patients had to undergo laser therapy again after 3 months, and 1 patient after 12 months. These 2 patients have now been free of recurrence for 7 and 9 months, respectively. In 1 of these cases renewed involvement of the external sphincter and prostatic urethra occurred. In none of the cases examined was a urethral stricture found. Initially feared complications, such as cavernitis, urethritis or induration of the corpus cavernosum, were not observed. The patient with condylomatous involvement of the external sphincter remained continent even after coagulation of this area.

Discussion

Since the introduction of neodymium-YAG laser coagulation for the treatment of bladder tumors [2, 10, 14], a technique has been available that is at least on par with, if not superior to, conventional snare resection, thanks to its advantages of contactless operation, circular sealing of afferent and efferent blood and lymph vessels, and an excellent depth effect [5]. With the further development and refinement of endoscopic equipment, we are now able to perform a large number of manipulations in the ureter under virtually the same conditions as in the bladder. Consequently, the concept of therapy for ureteral tumors must be reconsidered. Why should the same criteria not apply to ureteral tumors as to bladder tumors if they can be classified and destroyed by endoscopic means? That this is possible with endoscopic neodymium-YAG laser irradiation has been demonstrated [4]. Logically, the indication for nephroureterectomy, including the bladder outlet, can therefore be modified in accordance with the criteria leading to radical cystectomy. If necessary, in cases of invasion of deeper ureteral layers or a recurrence of a tumor with a low degree of differentiation, the radical operation can be repeated. With the reservations and criticism made necessary by the small number of cases, we believe that with the help of laser irradiation of ureteral tumors we have come a step closer to the goal of organ-preserving treatment [17].

On the basis of our results to date, we now feel justified in abandoning radical measures as a first step. After obtaining the exact classification of the tumor, laser irradiation does not preclude subsequent surgery. Worthy of note is the observation that no neighboring organs are injured and no strictures develop as late complications (fig. 2b). It should also be emphasized that the defect appears to be reepithelialized after just 2–3 weeks. The fact that the incidence of perforations in such a thin-walled organ is so low is probably due to the fact that irradiation is tangential. At the same time, however, tangential irradiation also presents a technical problem, since it means that only the distal side of the tumor is immediately accessible. For effective treatment, therefore, it is essential that the tumor be removed after coagulation, so that the so-called shadow areas can also be exposed.

The gratifying absence of strictures as a late complication is probably due to the fact that the integrity of the ureter is not compromised by laser coagulation.

From experimental studies on rat bladders we know that the architecture of the collagen fiber matrix is retained under laser irradiation [15]. Thus conditions are favorable for regeneration of the ureter. This is very likely the explanation for the absence of strictures so far.

Since all the techniques so far employed for the treatment of condylomatous involvement of deep ureteral sections have been associated with more or less high complication rates, the consideration that a relatively low rate of strictures may be expected with the neodymium-YAG laser led to its use for this indication as well. Moreover, excellent results have already been achieved with laser treatment of external condylomata.

The results obtained indicate that, even in the case of extreme involvement of the urethra, the old, sometimes mutilating methods should now be abandoned and that acceptable recurrence rates can be achieved.

The extent to which the cases described here were true recurrences or were primary condylomas that had been overlooked cannot be answered with certainty, since repeated movement of the instrument shaft might mechanically flatten small condylomas, thus rendering them unrecognizable.

In the afore-mentioned case in which additional involvement of the external sphincter and prostatic urethra were found on subsequent examination, the possibility must be considered of virus implantation by the irrigation stream or the instruments shaft. This has led to the requirement in our department that, in all cases of condylomatous disease, routine orientation urethrocystoscopy may be performed only with a laser light guide on standby, so that any condylomata found can be coagulated immediately without having to slide the instrument over the lesion. A decisive advantage of laser coagulation appears to be its architecture-preserving effect so that, at least in the case described in which coagulation of the sphincter area was performed, continence is maintained.

On the basis of our present knowledge, we advocate the following procedure for the adequate treatment of condyloma involvement deep within the urethra: (1) circumcision; (2) orientating cystoscopy with the laser on standby; (3) no catheterization; (4) short-term follow-up examinations, and (5) to prevent reinfection the partner should also be treated.

References

1 Böwering, R.; Hofstetter, A.; Frank, F.: Zerstörung von Tumoren der oberen Harnwege mit dem Neodym-Yag Laser, pp. 203–206 (Erdmann-Berger, Munich 1985).

2 Cormane, R.H.: Condylomata acuminata en podophylline. Ned. Tijdschr. Geneesk. *112:* 2305–2307 (1968).

3 Hofstetter, A.; Frank, F.: Der Neodym-YAG-Laser in der Urologie. Vol. 4: Medizinische Anwendung, pp. 43–55 (Editions Roche, Basel 1979).

4 Hofstetter, A.; Böwering, R.; Keiditsch, E.; Frank, F.: Zerstörung von Uretertumoren mit dem Neodym-YAG Laser, pp. 136–138 (Zuckschwerdt, Munich 1983).

5 Hofstetter, A.; Schilling, A.: Therapie und Rezidivprophylaxe oberflächlicher Harnblasenkarzinome, pp. 17–20 (Thieme, Stuttgart 1984).

6 Krebs, H.B.: The role of laser. Int. Conf. Laser Surg., Detroit 1983. Lasers Surg. Med. *3:* 134 (1983).

7 Lundquist, S.B.; Lindstedt, E.M.: Int. Conf. Laser Surg., Detroit 1983. Lasers Surg. Med. *3:* 152–153 (1983).

8 Montaldi, D.H.; Giambrone, J.P.; Gonrey, N.G.; Taefi, P.: Podophyllin poisoning associated with the treatment of condyloma acuminata: a case report. Am. J. Obstet. Gynec. *119:* 1130–1131 (1974).

9 Naidus, R.M.; Rodvien, R.; Mielke, C., Jr.: Colchicine toxicity: a multisystem disease. Archs intern. Med. *137:* 394–396 (1977).

10 Penzel, J.; Hofstetter, A.; Rothenberger, K.; Keiditsch, E.: Die Indikation für den Einsatz des Nd.-YAG Lasers in der Urologie, pp. 114–118 (Zuckschwerdt, Munich 1983).

11 Perez-Castro Ellendt, E.; Martinez-Pineiro, J.A.: Transurethrale Ureterpyeloskopie. Urologe A *20:* 258–260 (1981).

12 Rothenberger, K.; Hofstetter, A.; Geiger, M.; Böwering, R.; Frank, F.: Erfahrungsbericht über die externe Anwendung eines Nd.-YAG Lasers. Verh. dt. Ges. Urol. *31:* 241–242 (1979).

13 Schirren, C.G., Sr.: Schwere Allgemeinvergiftung nach örtlicher Anwendung von Podophyllinspiritus bei spitzen Condylomen. Hautarzt *17:* 321–322 (1966).

14 Staehler, G.; Hofstetter, A.; Schmiedt, E.; Rother, W.; Keiditsch, E.: Endoskopische Laser-Bestrahlung von Blasentumoren des Menschen. Fortschr. Med. *95:* 3–7 (1977).

15 Stern, J.; Zimmermann, J.; Frank, F.; Keiditsch, E.: Restitution der transmuralen Koagulationsnekrose nach Neodym-YAG-Laser-Bestrahlung, pp. 129–135 (Zuckschwerdt, Munich 1983).

16 Stoehr, G.P.; Peterson, A.L.; Taylor, W.J.: Systemic complications of cocal podophyllin therapy: a new operative technique. Soc. Med. *71:* 180–363 (1978).

17 Verst, S.A.: Conservative surgery in certain benign tumors of the ureter. J. Urol. *1945:* 53–97 (1945).

Dr. med. A. Schilling, Urologie, Klinikum Bogenhausen, Englschalkinger Strasse 77, D–8000 München 80 (FRG)

Eur. Urol. *12:* suppl. 1, pp. 34–36 (1986)

Value of the Neodymium-YAG Laser in the Therapy of Penile Carcinoma

K.H. Rothenberger

Department of Urology, Municipal Hospital Landshut, FRG

Key Words. Penile carcinoma · Neodymium-YAG laser · Devitalization · Tissue ablation

Abstract. Mutilation with associated functional losses characterizes current therapy of penile carcinoma. In addition, the recurrence rate is extremely high. Treatment with the neodymium-YAG laser provides a new therapy concept for T_1 and T_2 tumors, namely devitalization of all tumor cells with minimal tissue ablation. Following excision of the actual tumor, the base and margins of the excision are subjected to deep thermal denaturation without tissue removal. Over a mean observation period of 5 years, no local recurrence was found in 17 patients treated with this technique; only 1 patient died of metastases that remained undetected during primary staging.

Carcinoma of the penis is relatively rare in the USA and Europe. Occurring most often in the sixth decade of life, it accounts for 0.5–1.5% of all malignant diseases in men. As a rule, such carcinomas are of the squamous cell type and are usually highly differentiated and keratinizing. Their growth rate is relatively slow. Owing to the absence of pain and a sense of shame, penile carcinomas are often kept secret, even from the family physician. On the other hand, the initially non-exophytic growth of penile carcinomas may lead to misdiagnoses, such as balanitis, and prolonged incorrect therapy.

Tumor Staging

For any specific tumor therapy, precise staging is essential. Whereas the T stage of penile carcinoma is relatively easy to evaluate and metastases usually occur in more advanced stages, an assessment of the N stage is difficult. Lymph drainage from the penis is primarily via the criss-cross network of superficial inguinal lymph nodes and thence to the deep stations and lymph nodes along the iliac arteries to the aorta. Normal findings on palpation of the superficial inguinal region does not exclude the presence of lymphatic metastasis. Pedal lymphography also provides misleading information, frequently demonstrating the degenerative inflammatory changes of the inguinal lymph nodes. Probably not all the primary lymph nodes are demonstrated, so that an additional penile lymphography is required to image them. We therefore proceed as follows.

Following pedal lymphography the inguinal and iliacal lymph nodes are punctured with a fine needle under fluoroscopic control. If no tumor cells are found, surgical removal of the inguinal superficial lymph nodes, in particular the so-called sentinal lymph nodes (Cabanas), is performed. In the absence of evidence of tumor growth, radical lymphadenectomy is not performed because of the risk of subsequent chronic lymphedema. If tumor involvement is ascertained by means of the two aforementioned diagnostic procedures, therapeutic lymphadenectomy is attempted and adjuvant chemotherapy is usually instituted.

Neodymium-YAG Laser Therapy

When treating penile carcinoma we always perform radical circumcision. A tourniquet is then applied at the penis base and, under the bloodless conditions thus created, the macroscopically visible carcinoma is removed with a scalpel. Immediately afterward the excised area, including a 0.5-cm-wide margin, is treated with the laser. We aim to achieve a reproducible, homogeneous end deep necrosis to ensure complete devitalization of any remaining tumor cells with the neodymium-YAG laser. In this indication the laser is used purely for coagulation and not for ablation or cutting. The laser

1

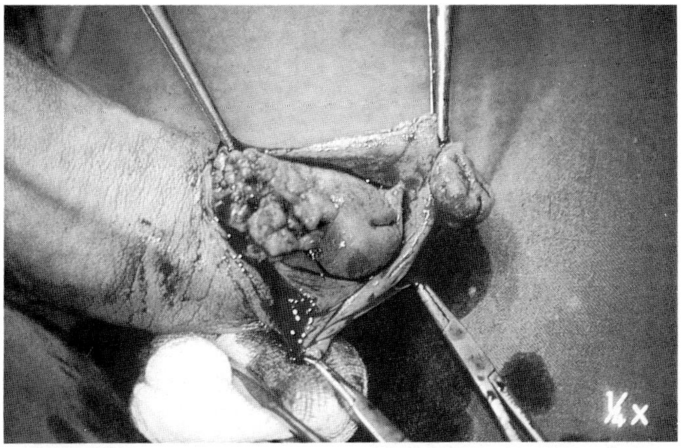

2

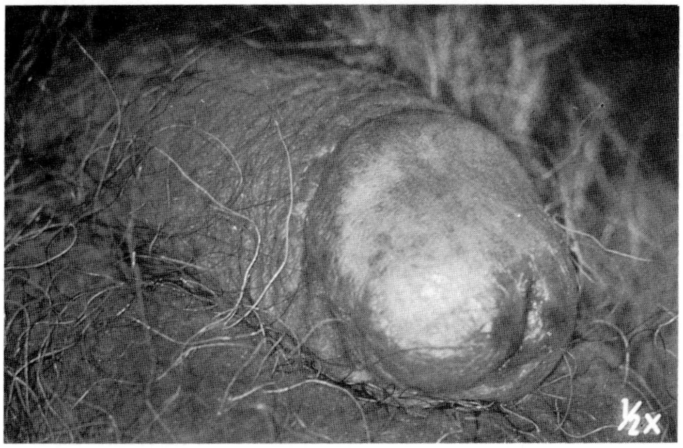

Fig. 1. A.S., 58 years old. Highly differentiated keratinizing squamous cell carcinoma.

Fig. 2. A.S., 58 years old. 3.5 years after laser therapy.

3

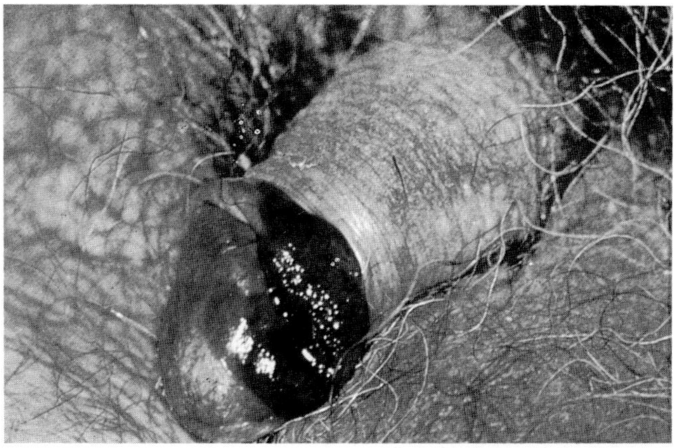

4

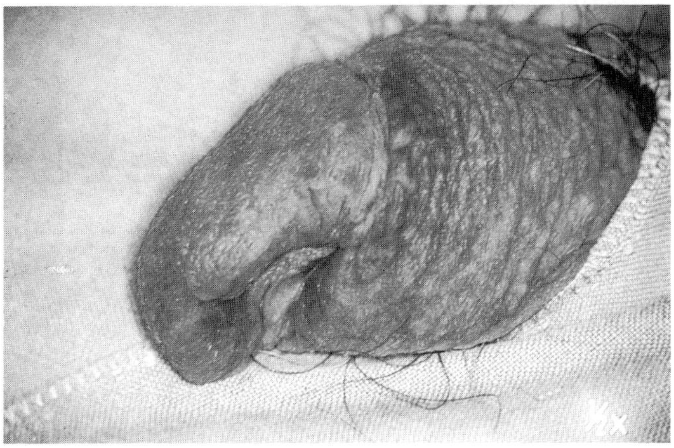

Fig. 3. K.S., 42 years old. Moderately differentiated, largely unkeratinized squamous cell carcinoma.

Fig. 4. K.S., 42 years old. 5 years after laser therapy.

light is transmitted through a flexible teflon-sheathed quartz-glass fiber light guide into a hand-held applicator with a focussing lens system. The latter permits the beam diameter to be changed, depending on the distance from the target. For the therapeutic effect of the laser on living tissue the product of laser output power and exposure time is decisive. In order to achieve the maximum necrosis depth of 3 mm without water cooling, a power output of 45 W must be applied for approximately 3 s. The depth of necrosis achieved can then be easily estimated on the basis of the white discoloration of the tissue surface. There is a point beyond which it is no longer possible to shorten the exposure time by increasing the laser power owing to superficial tissue changes, e.g. desiccation and carbonization. Carbonization increases tissue energy absorption by a factor of about 40, resulting in massive overheating of the surface and vaporization of the tissue. Thus, the actual depth of penetration is not increased. If the tissue surface is covered with blood, a similar effect occurs, since the absorption of laser energy by blood is also about 40 times greater than that of normal tissue. In this case the depth of penetration is even reduced.

If the tissue surface is cooled with water, rapid superficial tissue change is delayed, so that the coagulation temperature can also be attained in deeper zones without tissue ablation. In this manner necrosis depths of 6 mm can be achieved. Again, a white discoloration of the surface occurs; however, the small extent of visible white necrosis conveys the erroneous impression of an insufficent depth effect. In practice this means that when white discoloration just appears in conjunction with surface cooling, the spherical zone of necrosis has reached a depth of at least 4 mm. By scanning the beam line by line over the treatment area, an overlapping of the spherical necrosis zones with complete destruction of the surface results.

Specimens are then removed with the biopsy forceps to determine the therapeutic success. Despite the necrotization and the occurrence of typical distorsion patterns, histologic evaluation of the tissue is still possible.

If isolated bleeding should occur on release of the tourniquet, this can usually be readily controlled with the focussed laser.

The healing phase usually lasts 6–8 weeks, and the patient should be informed of this expressly prior to treatment. Daily chamomile penis baths promote clean healing. Initially, a loose bandage with Sofratüll® gauze or Nebacetin® ointment, for example, is recommended. Intensive follow-up with superficial tissue biopsies, when required, establishes the success of treatment.

Results (fig. 1–4)

So far we have treated 13 patients aged between 33 and 77 years with stage $T_1N_0M_0$ tumors, 6 patients aged between 42 and 86 years with $T_2N_0M_0$ carcinomas. In 2

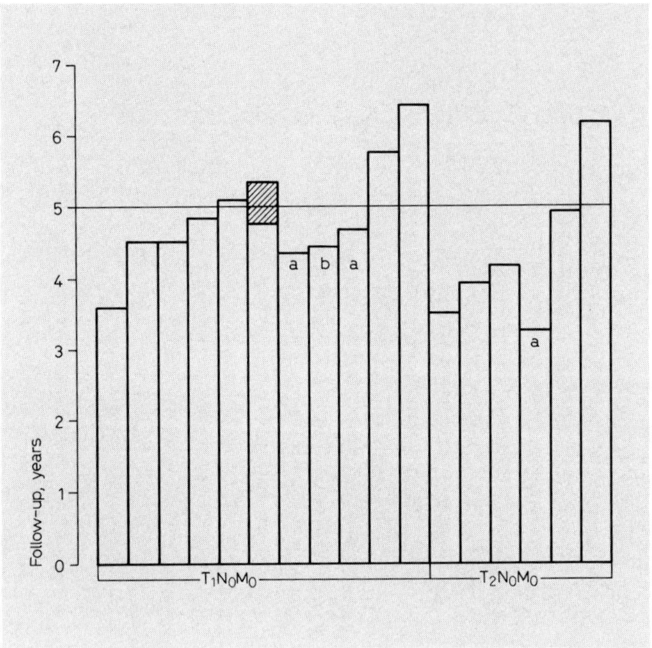

Fig. 5. Follow-up observation of 17 patients with penile carcinoma in stages T_1 to $T_2N_0M_0$. The hatched area of the sixth bar indicates the occurrence of Bowen's disease, which was also successfully treated with the laser.

of the stage $T_1N_0M_0$ patients we subsequently had to treat a carcinoma in situ with the laser within the first year. One patient developed Bowen's disease of the glans after 59 months, which was also successfully treated with the laser. In all of the other patients no pathological changes occurred in the area of the glans over an observation period of up to 6.5 years. Two patients of the $T_1N_0M_0$ group were treated this year (1985), and were not included in the further observation. Of the remaining 17 patients (fig. 5) with a follow-up observation period of between 43 and 77 months, 1 patient died of metastases of his penile carcinoma with no evidence of local tumor recurrence. Three other patients have died in the meantime of other diseases (esophageal carcinoma, bladder carcinoma, heart failure).

Two other patients with T_1 and T_2 carcinomas underwent therapeutic lymphadenectomy for lymph node metastases. Locally, no metastases occurred in either patient. One patient died of a bladder carcinoma after 59 months, the second patient lived for 62 months after primary therapy with no complaints and no evidence of disease.

Discussion

The results of conventional therapeutic approaches to cancer of the penis have so far not been very encouraging. Thus a recurrence rate of 40% is expected after local excision of the cancer [Hanash]. According to Gursel even partial amputation, i.e. removal of the tumor area 2 cm deep in healthy tissue, which results in considerable mutilation, is associated with a recurrence rate of 10%. For the same approach Salaverria reports a 5-year survival rate of only 77%! According to Pointon, high-voltage therapy is associated not only with strictures, burns and radionecrosis of the penis, but also a recurrence rate of 15%. Primary bleomycin therapy cannot be the therapy of choice since, despite initial hopes, Ichikawa reported a recurrence rate of 50%. In figure 5 the individual follow-up observations of the 17 patients with T_1 and T_2 tumors are represented. It can be seen that our report covers an average observation period of almost 5 years, during which we lost no patient to recurrent tumor. One patient was understaged. Even in a further case of a T_3 tumor (with involvement of the urethra), no local tumor recurrence was observed, although the patient died 34 months later of metastatic disease.

We believe that for treatment of penile carcinomas the described method of excision and neodymium-YAG laser therapy not only represents a true alternative, but is also the method of choice. The advantages of neodymium-YAG laser therapy of penile carcinoma are maintenance of miction and cohabitation functions, minimal cosmetic defects, no scarring with meatus constrictions, and an extremely low local recurrence rate.

References available from the author

Dr. med. K. Rothenberger,
Urologische Abteilung,
Städt. Krankenhaus Landshut,
Robert-Koch-Strasse 1,
D–8300 Landshut (FRG)

Eur. Urol. *12:* suppl. 1, pp. 37–38 (1986)

0302–2838/86/0127–0037$2.75/0

Experience with the Treatment of Localized Prostatic Carcinoma Using the Neodymium-YAG Laser

Preliminary Evaluation

Hans Olav Beisland, Sten Sander

Department of Surgery and Urology, Aker Hospital, Oslo, Norway

Key Words. Localized prostatic carcinoma · Neodymium-YAG laser irradiation · Preliminary evaluation

Abstract. Transurethral resection combined with subsequent neodymium-YAG laser irradiation of the prostatic capsule is a new modality for treating localized prostatic carcinoma. The technical procedure is simple, complications are few, and the treatment is well tolerated, even by high-risk patient. Clinical experience gained so far is promising, but follow-up has been too short to permit a definitive comparison with other treatment modalities.

Introduction

Prostatic tumor nodes are often located close to the capsule. Even when an extended transurethral resection (TUR) is carried out, remnants of tumor tissue are frequently left in the neighborhood of the capsule. The theoretical consideration behind the introduction of the neodymium-YAG laser to treat localized prostatic carcinoma was that any remaining tumor tissue could be destroyed by subsequent laser irradiation of the capsule. This idea was first described by Böwering et al. [1979], but only a few patients were treated. Since 1981 we have developed a technical procedure [Sander et al., 1982; Sander and Beisland, 1984] with which approximately 80 patients have been treated to date. The aim of this paper is to describe the technical procedure and to present a brief preliminary evaluation of the clinical results.

Material and Methods

Treatment is carried out in two separate steps. First TUR extending to the capsule and then, 3–5 weeks later, laser irradiation.

It is important that TUR be done by an experienced surgeon in order to leave an open cavity with smooth walls for the subsequent laser irradiation.

Laser irradiation is done under spinal anesthesia. The flexible light guide is introduced transurethrally through a 21-french panendoscope. Using the Albarran handle, the tip of the light guide can be angulated to almost 90 degrees. The prostatic cavity is systematically irradiated by slowly moving the beam. A laser power output setting of 45–50 W is selected, and the duration of each pulse does not exceed 4 s. The transurethral approach does not provide sufficient access for complete irradiation of the apical area. Consequently, the irradiation procedure is done by the additional use of a trocar cystoscope inserted suprapubically. Via this route the lower part of the cavity and the apical area can be properly irradiated.

To avoid the risk of damage to the rectum it is mandatory to interrupt the irradiation for 2–3 min at 10-pulse intervals when irradiating the posterior wall of the cavity [Beisland and Stranden, 1984]. The irrigation of the cavity with saline at room temperature must be continued during such an interrruption, in order to reduce the temperature. When irradiating the anterior and the lateral walls, there is no danger of the temperature increasing to hazardous levels.

The operating time is approximately 35 min. Postoperatively, a catheter is left in the bladder for 24 h. The patients are usually discharged 1 day after treatment.

For preoperative tumor staging, urethrocystoscopy, rectal palpation, and transrectal ultrasonography are carried out. The histological differentiation of the tumor is done on the basis of the TUR specimen in accordance with the WHO criteria. Investigations for possible distant metastases include blood analyses (sedimentation rate, hemoglobin), serum creatinine, acid and alkaline phosphatases, and bilirubin, chest X-ray, pelvic and lumbar bone films, and, where required, bone scan.

The present material comprises 63 patients who met the inclusion criteria, namely, tumors of stage $T_{1-2}N_xM_0$, irrespective of histological differentiation, and follow-up for more than 6 months.

Follow-up examinations were carried out at 3-month intervals during the first 2 years; thereafter every 6 months. The observation time ranged from 6 to 48 months (mean 22 months). Urethrocystoscopy was done 3 or 6 months postoperatively to verify proper epithelialization of the cavity. The local extension of the disease was evaluated by rectal palpation and transrectal ultrasonography. Whenever local tumor progression was suspected, thin-needle biopsies were obtained. Distant metastases were screened for by the same laboratory studies as preoperatively. X-rays and bone scan were performed after 6 months and at 1-year intervals thereafter.

The results have been divided into two groups: disease-free survivors and failures. Failure criteria are considered to be: development of distant metastases, persistent elevation of serum acid phosphatases, tumor progression beyond the prostatic capsule, or local recurrence of palpable tumor verified by biopsy to be a carcinoma.

Results

Preoperative complications did not occur. Postoperatively, acute cystitis, acute epididymitis, and spinal headache occurred in 3 patients requiring a prolongation of hospitalization. Late complications such as incontinence, strictures, or persisting urinary tract infection were not seen. At cystoscopy 3 or 6 monts after irradiation, all patients had a smoothly epithelialized and open prostatic cavity with no calcifications, ulcerations, or protrusions suspicious for tumor. Fifty-six patients are disease-free survivors. Clinically, they are doing well, their voiding pattern and sexual function being as seen after TUR alone. There has been no mortality, but treatment failed in 7 cases.

Three of these had recurrence of a local tumor node confirmed by biopsy to be a carcinoma of the same histological differentiation as the pretreatment tumor. Two of these also had elevated serum acid phosphatases and were, therefore, submitted to orchiectomy. The 3rd patient had only recurrence of a local tumor node, and he was again treated with TUR and laser.

Two patients had tumor progression beyond the prostatic capsule. One of them also developed distant metastases. The last 2 patients had distant metastases with no signs of local tumor recurrence.

Discussion

Prostatic carcinoma is often located in the apex [Byar et al., 1972]. Adequate irradiation of this region is, therefore, of great importance, and access to it can be effected only via the suprapubic trocar cystoscope. There have been no problems associated with the insertion of the trocar cystoscope.

Transrectal ultrasonography is essential for proper tumor staging and detection of tumor recurrence and progression during follow-up. Tumor involvement of the prostatic capsule or extention beyond the capsule can clearly be visualized on the ultrasonograms.

Staging lymphadenectomy has not been carried out, because our main purpose was to establish a method for controlling local disease. In this respect, the results obtained so far are promising and comparable to short-term results obtained with radiotherapy and/or interstitial implantation procedures. For evaluation of laser irradiation as radical treatment, staging lymphadenectomy should be carried out to ensure proper selection of the patients.

References

Beisland, H.O.; Stranden, E.: Rectal temperature monitoring during neodymium-YAG laser irradiation for prostatic carcinoma. Urol. Res. *12:* 257–259 (1984).

Böwering, R.; Hofstetter, A.; Keiditsch, E.; Frank, F.: Irradiation of prostatic carcinoma by neodymium-YAG laser. Optics Photonics appl. Med. *211:* 16–20 (1979).

Byar, D.P.; Mostofi, F.K.; Veterans Administration Cooperative Urological Research Group: Carcinoma of the prostate. Prognostic evaluation of certain pathological features in 208 radical prostatectomies. Cancer *30:* 5–13 (1972).

Sander, S.; Beisland, H.O.: Laser in the treatment of localized prostatic carcinoma. J. Urol. *132:* 280–281 (1984).

Sander, S.; Beisland, H.O.; Fossberg, E.: Neodymium-YAG laser treatment of prostatic cancer. Urol. Res. *10:* 85–86 (1982).

Dr. H.O. Beisland,
Department of Surgery and Urology,
Aker Hospital,
N-0514 Oslo (Norway)

Eur. Urol. *12:* suppl. 1, pp. 39–42 (1986)

0302–2838/86/0127–0039$2.75/0

Transrectal Ultrasonography before and after Neodymium-YAG Laser Irradiation of Localized Prostatic Carcinoma[1]

Hans Olav Beisland, Frode Lærum

Departments of Urology and Radiology, Aker Hospital, Oslo, Norway

Key Words. Localized prostatic carcinoma · Neodymium-YAG laser irradiation · Transrectal ultrasonography

Abstract. Transrectal ultrasonography was used to evaluate 54 patients with localized prostatic carcinoma treated with neodymium-YAG laser irradiation. Both pre- and postirradiation scans were obtained in 30 patients, while additional 24 cases were examined after laser irradiation only. The procedure represents a valuable contribution to proper preoperative staging and is mandatory for the follow-up of patients selected for this particular treatment. The shrinkage of the capsule is negligible after laser irradiation. No specific ultrasonic changes due to the laser effect are to be found. Abnormal parenchymal echoes and capsular irregularities are the major parameters indicating early recurrence of disease. The presence of malignancy must be confirmed by biopsy.

Introduction

Ultrasound has improved the diagnostic possibilities in prostatic disease. Scanning can be carried out transabdominally, transurethrally, or transrectally. Anatomical structures and pathological changes can be visualized, and the size of the gland can be measured accurately [1, 2]. Definitive ultrasonic criteria for distinguishing between benign and malignant lesions at an early stage have still not been established, and the diagnosis of carcinoma must be confirmed by biopsy [3, 4]. The main advantage of the method in patients with prostatic carcinoma is the possibility of proper staging of cytologically or histologically proven malignant disease. The transrectal scan permits accurate staging and case selection for radical treatment (T_1 and T_2), in addition to objective assessment of treatment response and possible local progression of disease.

On the basis of preliminary studies [5], transurethral resection (TUR) with subsequent laser irradiation of the prostatic capsule was introduced as a means of treating localized prostatic carcinoma [6]. The rationale of this treatment is that if the bulk of prostatic tissue is removed by TUR, it should be possible to destroy any remaining carcinomatous tissue in the capsule area by laser irradiation.

The purpose of the present report is to evaluate transrectal ultrasonography as a preoperative and follow-up procedure and to correlate the ultrasonographic and clinical findings. In addition, we looked for possible specific ultrasonographic features of the laser effect.

Material and Methods

Patients with localized prostatic carcinoma (stage T_1 and T_2) with no distant metastases are candidates for combined treatment with TUR and laser. The treatment is carried out in two separate steps: first TUR extending to the capsule and then laser irradiation 3–5 weeks later.

Of 64 patients investigated ultrasonically, 25 were excluded from radical treatment because of advanced tumor stage. Of 39 patients

[1] Specially invited supplementary contribution to article pp. 37–38.

Table I. Survey of ultrasonic results before and after neodymium-YAG laser irradiation of localized prostatic carcinoma

	Before laser	After laser		
		3–6 months	6–12 months	12–24 months
	(n = 39)	(n = 32)	(n = 25)	(n = 25)
Prostatic capsule				
Normal	38	25	21	23
Irregular	1	7	4	2
Prostatic parenchyma				
Normal echoes	36	29	19	22
Suspicious foci	3	3	6	3
Prostatic cavity				
Small	9	9	7	13
Large	30	23	18	12
Seminal vesicles				
Normal	34	30	21	21
Not visualized	5	2	4	4
Calcifications	26	18	19	17
Mean maximal transverse diameter of capsule, mm	46	44	43	44

Table II. Correlation between ultrasonic findings in the prostatic capsule and in the prostatic parenchyma after neodymium-YAG laser irradiation of localized prostatic carcinoma

	Prostatic capsule	
	irregular (n = 13)	normal (n = 69)
Prostatic parenchyma		
Suspicious foci (n = 12)	6	6
Normal echoes (n = 70)	7	63

treated by laser irradiation, 30 have been followed up with ultrasonography. In addition, 24 patients have been examined ultrasonically after laser irradiation only. This is because laser therapy was established 1½ years before the present ultrasound technique became available at our department. Thus the material consists of preirradiation ultrasonograms of 39 and follow-up ultrasonograms of 54 patients. Most of the preirradiation examinations were performed after TUR. The results obtained 3–6, 6–12, and 12–24 months after laser irradiation are evaluated separately.

Laser irradiation was carried out in accordance with a standardized procedure [7] using a neodymium-YAG laser (MBB, Munich-Ottobrunn, FRG). With a laser power output setting of 45–50 W, the prostatic capsule was systematically irradiated by overlapping pulses of 4 s duration. A combination of transurethral and suprapubic approaches was used to achieve complete access to all parts of the cavity.

The ultrasonographic examinations were done with an ATL 300® (Advanced Technology Laboratories Inc., USA) ultrasound machine and a 90-degree prototype sector probe (No. 202) designed for frequencies of 5.0 and 7.5 MHz for transversal rectal examination. Only the 7.5-MHz frequency was used. The rectal probe is designed with a pistol-handle, 11.5-cm shaft with a diameter of 1.5 cm for introduction into the rectum. A rubber condom applied over the shaft and an angiographic catheter was fixed with rubber bands 4–5 cm from the tip. By injecting 30–60 ml saline through the angiographic catheter, a balloon at the tip of the probe was caused to distend, securing contact to the rectal mucosa and establishing the proper distance to the structures to be scanned. To avoid air bubbles in the balloon, a small amount of methylpolysiloxane (Minifom®, 'Tika') was added to the fluid to reduce the surface tension. The patients were examined in a left decubitus position. The prostatic gland was systematically scanned along a sagittal and two oblique axes.

The following parameters served for evaluation of the ultrasonograms: the maximal transverse diameter of the capsule, the integrity of the prostatic capsule, visualization of the seminal vesicles, focal parenchymal abnormalities and calcifications. The size of the cavity was not measured exactly, but estimated to be 'small' or 'large'. Suspicious ultrasonic findings during follow-up were investigated by thin-needle biopsy.

Results

A survey of the results is given in table I. Before laser irradiation 1 patient had suspected capsule breach and a suspicious parenchymal focus. TUR was repeated, but no residual carcinoma was found in the specimens. Two more patients had ultrasonically suspected small foci which, however, were not detectable after irradiation, and there were no clinical signs of recurrent disease.

A correlation between capsular irregularities and focal abnormalities indicating possible disease after laser irradiation is shown in table II. The 20 ultrasonograms were obtained from 13 patients. Two patients with both irregular capsule and parenchymal foci had positive biopsies. One of them was the patient mentioned above who had the same changes prior to laser treatment. In 3 cases with suspicious parenchymal foci only, positive biopsies were found. Negative biopsies were obtained in all cases of capsular irregularities only. Biopsies were not carried out routinely in patients with both normal capsule and parenchymal echoes, but only in cases with a particularly hard consistency of the capsule on rectal palpation.

In 5 pretreatment and 10 posttreatment scans, the seminal vesicles were not detectable by ultrasound. In 2 patients only, nonvisualization of the vesicles correlated with recurrent disease, both having a combination of capsule involvement and abnormal parenchymal echoes.

A minor decrease in maximal transverse diameter of the capsule was demonstrated 3–6 months after laser treatment. Additional shrinkage did not occur during follow-up (table I).

Before laser irradiation 23% of the prostatic cavities were estimated to be small. The mean weight of tissue resected from glands with small cavities was 17 g (range 8–36) as compared with 28 g (range 14–76) from resections leaving large cavities. 12–24 months after laser irradiation 52% of the cavities were estimated to be small.

Calcifications in the prostate were seen in 67% of the patients before treatment and in 66% at follow-up. In 25 patients excluded from laser irradiation because of advanced tumor stage, 84% had calcifications within the gland. Among 30 patients investigated both before and after laser irradiation, 5 patients had calcifications before but not after, while 4 patients had calcifications after but not before treatment. Before treatment 42% of the patients with calcifications had moderately or poorly differentiated carcinomas (WHO II–III), while 77% of the patients without calcifications had well-differentiated carcinomas (WHO I). 78% of WHO II–III tumors demonstrated calcifications, as did 60% of WHO I tumors.

Discussion

Ultrasonography permits visualization of the anterolateral aspects of the prostate that are not accessible to digital palpation. Tumors and capsular breach may well be situated in these areas [8].

The neodymium-YAG laser light penetrates 5–6 mm into biological tissue. The transformation of light energy into heat causes deep homogeneous coagulation of all structures [9]. The framework of tissue is kept intact during the period of restitution, and, therefore, the risk of late perforation of a hollow organ is minimal [10]. Necrotic tissue is gradually replaced by fibrotic scar tissue with remarkable little shrinkage [11]. Owing to this property, only a slight decrease in the maximal transverse diameter of the capsule can be demonstrated after laser irradiation. Any decrease in diameter or volume of the gland is, therefore, a poor indicator of treatment efficacy, in contrast with cases treated conservatively by endocrine procedures or radiotherapy [12, 13].

The number of prostatic cavities, estimated to be small, increased with time after laser irradiation. This phenomenon is also seen after conventional TUR of the prostate. It is also known that the resection cavity is occupied by a variable echo pattern [2].

An aim of this study was to examine whether laser-coagulated tissue could be distinguished from nonirradiated tissue ultrasonically, and the depth of the laser effect thus visualized. Early postoperative scans detected histologically benign capsule irregularities more frequently as compared with later examinations. This may indicate that laser treatment induces reversible ultrasonic changes. No constant specific laser-related changes were found, however.

The nonvisualization of the seminal vesicles was related to recurrence and progression of the disease in 2 patients only. Failure to demonstrate the seminal vesicles ultrasonically in prostatic carcinoma does not necessarily signify their malignant infiltration [14]. Ultrasonic involvement of the vesicles is probably of later occurrence than capsule involvement and appearance of abnormal echoes. In 48% of patients excluded from laser treatment because of advanced tumor stage, vesicle involvement was detected.

The focal abnormalities were not grouped according to echogenicity, since neither echoic, hypoechoic, nor mixed echoes are specific for malignancy [15]. All glands with abnormal parenchymal echoes were examined bioptically with the fine-needle technique. Five out of 13 patients with abnormal foci had a positive biopsy, and these cases were defined as true recurrences with a need for additional treatment. The origin of the foci not proven to be carcinoma is unknown, but these patients are being followed with particular care.

No typical pattern of prostatic calcification is associated with carcinoma [3, 16]. Only few patients had microcalcifications, and this was not related to tumor recurrence. Increased calcification after laser irradiation could not be demonstrated, and calcifications on the inside surface of the cavity were not detected in any patients by urethrocystoscopy carried out 3–6 months after treatment. There was no correlation between calcification and the presence of focal abnormalities or capsule irregularities. The observation that calcifications are more frequent in poorly and moderately differentiated carcinomas as compared with well-differentiated carcinomas, may be a coincidence.

Transrectal ultrasonography represents a diagnostic advantage in prostatic carcinoma. The whole gland can be visualized and proper staging achieved. This is of importance for selecting the patients for optimal treatment and for adequate follow-up. The investigation procedure is simple and, with some experience, can be carried out quickly and safely, also in the outpatient department. This study confirms that suspicious ultrasonic findings need to be confirmed by biopsy.

References

1 Bartsch, G.; Egender, G.; Hübscher, H.; Rohr, H.: Sonometrics of the prostate. J. Urol. *127:* 1119–1121 (1982).
2 Hastak, S.M.; Gammelgaard, J.; Holm, H.H.: Transrectal ultrasonic volume determination of the prostate – a preoperative and postoperative study. J. Urol. *127:* 1115–1118 (1982).
3 Harada, K.; Igari, D.; Tanahashi, Y.: Gray scale transrectal ultrasonography of the prostate. J. clin. Ultrasound *7:* 45–49 (1979).
4 Hastak, S.M.; Gammelgaard, J.; Holm, H.H.: Ultrasonically guided transperineal biopsy in the diagnosis of prostatic carcinoma. J. Urol. *128:* 69–71 (1982).
5 Böwering, R.; Hofstetter, A.; Keiditsch, E.; Frank, F.: Irradiation of prostatic carcinoma by neodymium-YAG laser. Optics Photonics appl. Med. *211:* 16–20 (1979).
6 Sander, S.; Beisland, H.O.; Fossberg, E.: Neodymium-YAG laser treatment of prostatic cancer. Urol. Res. *10:* 85–86 (1982).
7 Sander, S.; Beisland, H.O.: Laser in the treatment of localized prostatic carcinoma. J. Urol. *132:* 280–281 (1984).
8 Brooman, P.J.C.; Griffiths, G.J.; Roberts, E.; Peeling, W.B.; Evans, K.: Per rectal ultrasound in the investigation of prostatic disease. Clin. Radiol. *32:* 669–676 (1981).
9 Halldórsson, T.: Biophysical fundamentals and instrumentation for the endovesical Nd:YAG laser application. Urologe A *20:* 293–299 (1981).
10 Keiditsch, E.: Histological changes following endovesical neodymium-YAG laser irradiation. Urologe A *20:* 300–304 (1981).
11 Hofstetter, A.; Frank, F.: The neodymium-YAG laser in Urology (Hoffmann-La Roche, Basel 1980).
12 Resnick, M.I.; Willard, J.W.; Boyce, W.H.: Transrectal ultrasonography in the evaluation of patients with prostatic carcinoma. J. Urol. *124:* 482–484 (1980).
13 Carpentier, P.J.; Schroeder, F.H.; Blom, J.H.M.: Transrectal ultrasonography in the follow-up of prostatic carcinoma patients. J. Urol. *128:* 742–746 (1982).
14 Peeling, W.B.; Griffiths, G.J.: Imaging of the prostate by ultrasound. J. Urol. *132:* 217–224 (1984).
15 Rifkin, M.D.; Kurtz, A.B.; Choi, H.Y.; Goldberg, B.B.: Endoscopic ultrasonic evaluation of the prostate using a transrectal probe: prospective evaluation and acoustic characterization. Radiology *149:* 265–271 (1983).
16 Harada, K.; Tanahashi, Y.; Igari, D.; Numata, I.; Orikasa, S.: Clinical evaluation of inside echo patterns in grey scale prostatic echography. J. Urol. *124:* 216–220 (1980).

Dr. H.O. Beisland,
Department of Surgery and Urology,
Aker Hospital,
N–0514 Oslo (Norway)

Eur. Urol. *12:* suppl. 1, pp. 43–46 (1986)

0302–2838/86/0127–0043$2.75/0

Integral Laser – Photodynamic Treatment of Multifocal Bladder Carcinoma Photosensitized by Hematoporphyrin Derivative

D. Jocham[a], *E. Schmiedt*[a], *R. Baumgartner*[b], *E. Unsöld*[b]

[a] Urologische Klinik und Poliklinik (Direktor: Prof. *E. Schmiedt*) der Ludwig-Maximilians-Universität, Klinikum Grosshadern, München, BRD; [b] Zentrales Laser-Labor der GSF-Neuherberg, Abteilung für angewandte Optik (Leiter: Prof. *W. Waidelich*), Neuherberg, BRD

Key Words. Multifocal bladder carcinoma · Carcinoma in situ · Photodynamic therapy · Hematoporphyrin derivative · Diffusion medium

Abstract. Intravenously administered hematoporphyrin derivative photosensitizes tumorous bladder tissue which can then be destroyed selectively by irradiation with red laser light (630 nm). After experimentally developing a concept since 1978 (light diffusion medium, special bladder catheter) to expose the bladder to the therapeutically effective red laser light, the integral photodynamic therapy is meanwhile performed clinically. The experience gained so far demonstrates that especially the multifocal carcinoma in situ up till now difficult to be detected endoscopically represents a new domain for the integral photodynamic therapy.

The treatment of certain types of bladder tumor still represents a special challenge for the urologist. Photodynamic therapy (PDT) following intravenously applied hematoporphyrin derivative (HpD) seems to be a new treatment modality for superficial bladder cancer, capable of supplementing, or in some cases even supplanting, established therapeutic methods. This therapeutic technique – a tissue-destroying photodynamic process – is based on the use of the photosensitizing substance HpD.

HpD shows the following properties: (1) tumor-specific deposition; (2) photosensitizing effects; (3) fluorescence; (4) no toxicity or carcinogenicity, and (5) as a side effect transient photosensitization of the skin and mucosa to sunlight.

HpD is a mixture of various porphyrin complexes. Following intravenous administration (in clinical use 1.0–2.5 mg/kg body weight) HpD is deposited in bladder tumor tissue of various degrees of differentiation (as well as in tumor tissue of numerous other organ systems) in substantially higher concentrations (factor 2–5) than in normal tissue. Also in comparison with tumor tissue, healthy tissue generally exhibits a more rapid clearance of the substance, even in the case of low HpD deposition down to tissue levels which are no longer photodynamically relevant. However, even after 30 days, HpD can still be detected in small concentrations in normal bladder tissue by means of sensitive fluorescence techniques, whereas other normal tissues, (e.g., liver, muscle, tongue) are completely free of HpD at this time. The causes underlying the differing pharmacokinetics of HpD in tumor and normal tissue are still unknown.

If HpD-photosensitized tissue is exposed to light of a wavelength which photodynamically excites the porphyrin molecule, cytotoxic processes may be induced in the tissue, depending on the power density and radiation dose, resulting in destruction of the tissue. If the exposure takes place at a time at which only tumor tissue still contains high concentrations of HpD, circumscribed areas of tumor destruction can be achieved. Experimental and clinical studies have shown that bladder tumor tissue, including carcinoma in situ (CIS), can be photodynamically destroyed [11, 15].

Initial reports on the PDT of human bladder tumors go back to 1976, when Kelly and Snell [16] reported on the successful photodynamic destruction of bladder tumor tissue by means of endoscopically controlled exposure to a mercury vapor lamp following the intravenous administration of HpD. In the meantime a lot of work has been done in the field of PDT for bladder carcinoma.

1 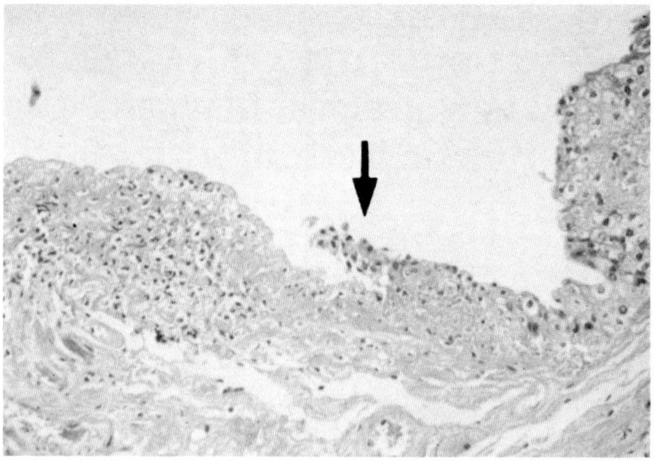

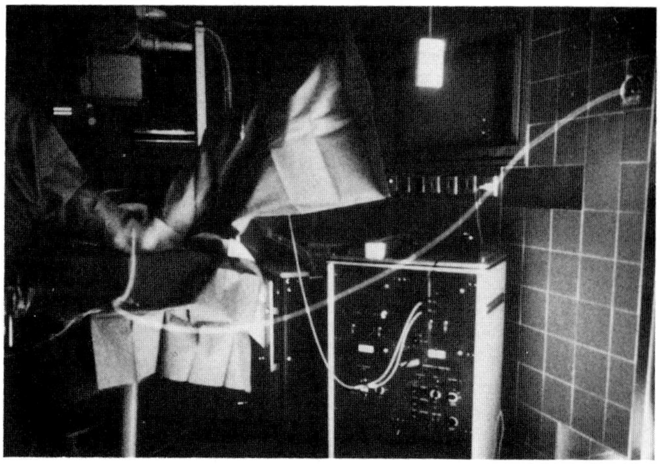
3

2 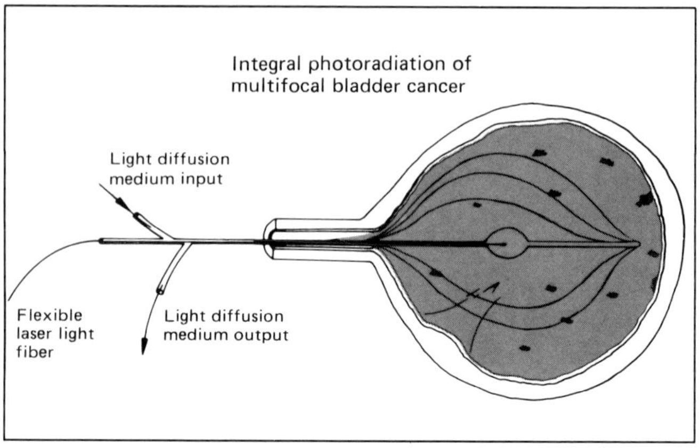

Fig. 1. Experimental superficial bladder carcinoma, PDT-related tumor destruction within the field of irradiation, on the left of the arrow. No change of tumor tissue in the light-protected area on the right of the arrow.

Fig. 2. Scheme of integral PDT. The bladder is irrigated by a milky solution which allows diffuse light irradiation of all regions of the bladder. The fiber tip is positioned in the center of the bladder using a special catheter. Multifocal tumor tissue is destroyed photodynamically by the photodynamic process.

Fig. 3. Clinical application of PDT in the treatment of multifocal CIS. Light from the laser – operated in a separate room – is transmitted through a flexible light fiber to the patient's bladder.

On the basis of our own experience and reports from other working groups [3–6, 8–10, 15, 18, 20], and taking into consideration the depth of infiltration, PDT appears justified only for CIS and T1 and T2 tumors. In our opinion, the excellent therapeutic response of hitherto poorly treatable CIS, as observed, among others, by Benson et al. [4], Benson [6], and Jocham et al. [15], makes this type of tumor the main indication for PDT.

In view of the special clinical picture of the common multifocal carcinoma at various developmental stages, irradiation of endoscopically visible bladder tumors did not appear to offer advantages over other forms of therapy. Moreover, only with the development of high-power lasers as a source of therapeutically effective light, in conjunction with special irradiation techniques, were the requirements met for the use of PDT for treatment of the common multifocal carcinoma at various stages of development.

Experimental studies we have carried out since 1978 demonstrate the possibility of reproducible selective tumor destruction (fig. 1) following intravenous application of HpD and irradiation with red light (630 nm) at a time when the porphyrins have been adequately cleared from normal tissue [10–14].

A precondition for achieving satisfactory therapeutic results was – as extensive preliminary investigations had shown – the development of suitable irradiation modalities. The goal was the exposure of multifocal bladder carcinoma in its entirety, including the parts of the tumor that cannot be detected endoscopically [11].

After experimentally testing numerous techniques, we found the use of a light diffusion medium to be an effective approach that has since been confirmed clinically. The end of the laser light guide is positioned in the center of the bladder with the aid of a special bladder catheter designed by us. This permits irradiation without endoscopic control which could not be performed expediently within the milky solution (fig. 2). The patients we have treated by integral PDT usually present with a multiple recurrent multifocal G 2-3 carcinoma and histologically

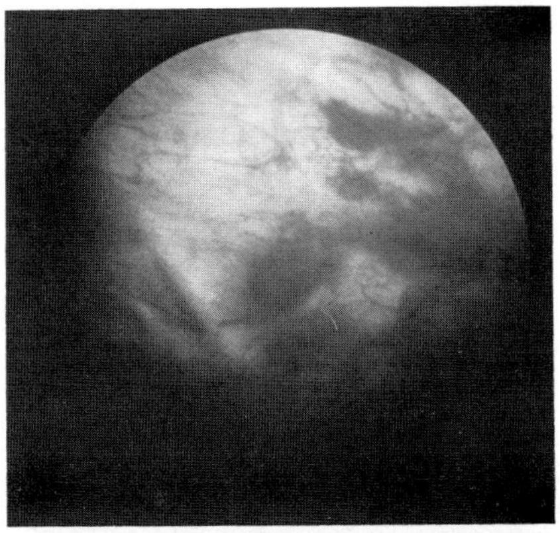
4

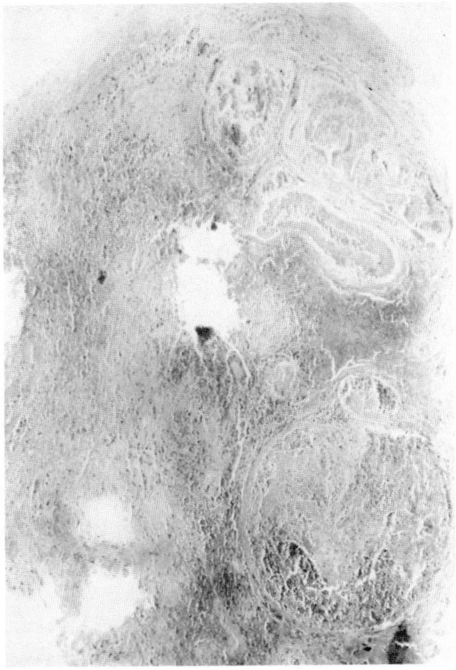
5

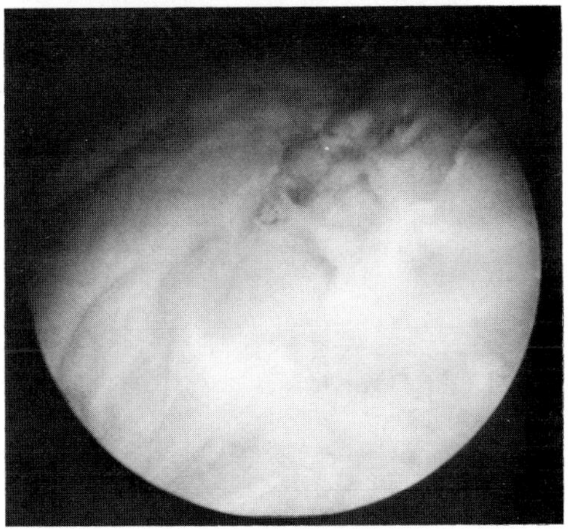
6

Fig. 4. Tumor-specific hemorrhagic necrosis of CIS in a part of the bladder which looked normal before PDT.

Fig. 5. Histology of tumor necrosis after PDT: eosinophilic inflammation.

Fig. 6. Almost total destruction of bladder mucosa following PDT (special case).

proven CIS. 50–96 h after intravenous injection of 2 mg HpD/kg body weight integral PDT is performed.

Figures 3 and 4 illustrate 1 typical case. Figure 3 demonstrates the situation during exposure – the light guide in the special catheter and the bladder irrigated by the light-scattering medium and irradiated by laser light at a wavelength of 630 nm.

With respect to the radiation dose, 15–70 J of energy per square centimeter of bladder wall surface are delivered over a period of 10–130 min. In the case demonstrated, no exophytic tumors were to be found at a cystoscopic examination performed routinely on the 5th postoperative day. In their place hemorrhagic mucosal zones of varying degree were seen (fig. 4). These hemorrhagic areas can sometimes also be found in bladder regions that are thought to be healthy before treatment. However, it should be stressed that there are also numerous areas which appear normal after therapy. Biopsies from these areas usually show histopathologically normal urothelium. Histologic examination of hemorrhagic areas typically reveals tumor necrosis with pronounced eosinophilic inflammatory reaction (fig. 5). In most cases, intact residual tumor tissue is not found in any of the numerous follow-up biopsies. Such good results can be reported for 4 out of 5 cases. It must be stated that following PDT patients complain of pollakisuria and a burning sensation on micturition for at least 3 weeks, sometimes much longer. Finally, patients become free of symptoms. It has to be stated that in 1 case with a pre-existing bladder capacity of only 120 cm^3 following 20 transurethral resections done elsewhere, open surgery of bladder perforation, and X-ray irradiation of bladder cancer, affection of nearly all areas of bladder mucosa and some further shrinkage of the bladder following PDT were observed. Figure 6 demonstrates the endoscopic appearance of necrotic bladder mucosa. Finally, it became necessary to perform cystectomy in this case. There was no tumor tissue found at the site of a pretreatment G II multifocal tumor including CIS. There was also proof of some remaining areas of normal urothelium.

Discussion

There is no doubt that superficial bladder tumor tissue can be effectively destroyed by PDT. Besides exhibiting merely a certain expediency, any new therapeutic method must also stand up to comparison with alternative techniques. An effective reduction in the recurrence rate of bladder carcinoma can, in our opinion, be reliably evaluated only after observation periods of more than 2 years. Only by means of randomized studies using local cytostatics or BCG can the efficacy of photodynamic bladder tumor therapy be assessed. In the future, urologists using PDT will have to address themselves to this painstaking task, and standardized therapeutic modalities will have to be observed.

In view of the as yet limited clinical experience gained to date, the significance of the side effects observed in particular cases – in particular damage to large bladder parts and associated shrinkage of the bladder – is unclear.

A possible explanation for this might be individually inadequate HpD clearance of normal bladder sections, or extensive tumor invasion and a corresponding therapeutic reaction.

The choice of treatment time following HpD administration and radiation dose – at present largely empirical – will be optimized only with greater clinical experience.

Despite this reservation, experience gained so far suggests that PDT may be able, reliably and effectively, to close a decisive therapeutic gap in the treatment of bladder cancer, in particular CIS.

References

1 Baghdassarian, R.; Wright, M.W.; Vaughn, S.A.; Bern, M.W.; Martin, D.C.; Will, A.G.: The use of lipid emulsion as an intravesical medium to disperse light in the potential treatment of bladder tumors. J. Urol. *133:* 126 (1985).

2 Baumgartner, R.; Stepp, H.; Ruprecht, L.; Unsöld, E.; Jocham, D.: Experimental study on fluorescence diagnosis of bladder cancer; in Jori, Perria, Photodynamic therapy of tumors and other diseases, p. 260 (Libreria Progetto Editore, Padova 1985).

3 Benson, R.C., Jr.; Kinsey, J.H.; Cortese, D.A.; Farrow, G.M.; Utz, D.C.: Treatment of transitional cell carcinoma of the bladder with hematoporphyrin derivative phototherapy. J. Urol. *130:* 1090 (1983).

4 Benson, R.C., Jr.; Farrow, G.M.; Kinsey, J.H.; Cortese, D.A.; Zincke, H.; Utz, D.C.: Detection and localization of in situ carcinoma of the bladder with hematoporphyrin derivative. Mayo Clin. Proc. *57:* 548 (1982).

5 Benson, R.C., Jr.: Photochemotherapy of bladder cancer; in Spitzky, Karrer, Proc. 13th Int. Congr. of Chemotherapy, Vienna 1983, pp. 31–35.

6 Benson, R.C., Jr.: Treatment of diffuse transitional cell carcinoma in situ by whole bladder hematoporphyrin derivative photodynamic therapy. J. urol. *134:* 675 (1985).

7 Goetz, A.; Feyh, J.; Schneckenburger, H.; Conzen, P.; Jocham, D.; Unsoeld, E.: Quantitative in vivo measurements of photofrin II in tumor and adjacent tumor-free tissues; in Jori, Perria, Photodynamic therapy of tumors and other diseases (Libreria Progetto Editore, Padova 1985).

8 Hisazumi, H.; Misaki, I.; Miyoshi, U.: Photoradiation therapy of bladder tumors. J. Urol. *130:* 685 (1983).

9 Hisazumi, H.; Miyoshi, N.; Naito, K.; Misaki, T.: Whole bladder wall photoradiation therapy for carcinoma in situ of the bladder: a preliminary report. J. Urol. *131:* 884 (1984).

10 Jocham, D.; Staehler, G.; Chaussy, Ch.; Hammer, C.; Löhrs, U.: Laserbehandlung von Blasentumoren nach Photosensibilisierung mit Hämatoporphyrin-Derivat. Urologe A *20:* suppl., p. 340 (1981).

11 Jocham, D.; Staehler, G.; Chaussy, Ch.; Löhrs, U.; Unsöld, E.: C.E. Alken Preis 1983: Integrale Photoradiotherapie des Blasenkarzinoms nach tumorselektiver Photosensibilisierung mit Hämatoporphyrin-Derivat (HpD). Akt. Urol. *15:* 109 (1984).

12 Jocham, D.; Unsöld, E.: Photodynamic therapy of bladder tumors; in Jori, Perria, Photodynamic therapy of tumors and other diseases, p. 290 (Libreria Progetto Editore, Padova 1985).

13 Jocham, D.; Staehler, G.; Chaussy, Ch.; Dietrich, R.; Weinsheimer, W.; Löhrs, E.: Integrale Photoradiotherapie des multifokalen Blasenkarzinoms. Verh. dt. Ges. Lasermed., 2. Tagung (Erdmann-Brenger, München 1985).

14 Jocham, D.; Staehler, G.; Chaussy, Ch.; Löhrs, U.; Unsöld, E.: Experimentelle und erste klinische Erfahrungen mit der integralen Photoradiotherapie des multifokalen Blasenkarzinoms und des Carcinoma in situ nach tumorselektiver Photosensibilisierung mit Hämatoporphyrin-Derivat. Helv. chir. Acta *52:* 469 (1985).

15 Jocham, D.; Staehler, G.; Baumgartner, R.; Unsöld, E.: Die integrale photodynamische Therapie beim multifokalen Blasenkarzinom – erste klinische Erfahrungen, Urologe A 316–319 (1985).

16 Kelly, J.F.; Snell, M.E.: Hematoporphyrin derivative: a possible aid in the diagnosis and therapy of carcinoma of the bladder. J. Urol. *115:* 150 (1976).

17 Reiner, S.; Stepp, H.; Baumgartner, R.; Jocham, D.; Kummermehr, J.; Unsöld, E.: A Murine tumor test model for photosensitizing agents; in Jori, Perria, Photodynamic therapy of tumors and other diseases, p. 228 (Libreria Progetto Editore, Padova 1985).

18 Rothauge, C.F.; Röttger, P.; Kraushaar, J.; Kracht, J.; Nöske, H.D.: Die Phototherapie des Blasenkarzinoms im Licht der Histologie. Diagnostik Intensivther. *8:* 17 (1983).

19 Schneckenburger, H.; Pauker, F.; Unsöld, E.; Jocham, D.: Intracellular distribution and retention of the fluorescent components of photofrin II. Photobiochem. Photobiophys. *10:* 61 (1985).

20 Tsuchiya, A.; Obara, U.; Miwa, M.; Oi, T.; Kato, H.; Hayata, Y.: Hematoporphyrin derivative and laser photoradiation in the diagnosis and treatment of bladder cancer. J. Urol. *130:* 79 (1983).

Dr. D. Jocham,
Urologische Klinik und Poliklinik,
Ludwig-Maximilians-Universität,
Marchioninistrasse 15, D–8000 München 70 (FRG)

Eur. Urol. *12:* suppl. 1, pp. 47–53 (1986)

Integral Photoradiation Therapy of Multifocal Bladder Tumors

Ralph C. Benson, Jr.

Department of Urology, Mayo Clinic and Mayo Foundation, Rochester, Minn., USA

Key Words. Hematoporphyrin derivative · Laser · Transitional cell carcinoma · Bladder cancer · Photodynamic therapy

Abstract. Focal and diffuse hematoporphyrin derivative (HpD) photodynamic therapy was used for the treatment of resistant transitional cell carcinoma in situ (Tis) in 30 patients. Patients were given HpD intravenously followed by either focal light irradiation (630 nm) or diffuse bladder irradiation via a light bulb fiber. The light source was an argon ion pumped dye laser circulating rhodamine B dye. All patients were followed with periodic cystoscopic examinations, bladder biopsies, and urine cytologic examinations. All of the 15 patients who underwent focal therapy had biopsy and cytologic evidence of disappearance of the lesion in the treated area at the 3-month follow-up cystoscopic examination. Eight patients have experienced one or more recurrent lesions either in the treated area or in distant areas, and in each the recurrence was successfully treated with HpD photodynamic therapy. Eight of the 11 patients with diffuse Tis have returned for their 3-month follow-up evaluation, and all demonstrated disappearance of tumor (3 of these 8 patients have subsequently developed focal recurrent Tis). Four patients had diffuse Tis plus T_a lesions (2 patients) or T_2 lesions (2 patients), and all had disappearance of the Tis, but persistance of the T_a or T_2 disease. We conclude that HpD photodynamic therapy appears effective in the treatment of resistant Tis.

Transitional cell carcinoma in situ (Tis) of the urinary bladder is usually treated with conservative measures such as fulguration and intravesical chemotherapy. The majority of the patients, however, will experience disease recurrence, and the only effective treatment for recurrent resistant Tis of the bladder has been cystectomy and urinary diversion. The necessity for such a radical approach has been demonstrated, yet the use of surgery of such magnitude and consequence for superficial cancer is unfortunate. For this reason many investigators have actively sought alternative treatment approaches.

Absorption of light by one molecule leading to the chemical alteration of another molecule is termed a photosensitized reaction. The light-absorbing molecule is termed the photosensitizer, and the other molecule is termed the substrate of the reaction. Photosensitizers, light, and oxygen have been known for years to be toxic to cells [1]. On the basis of this principle, a new approach to the treatment of various malignant lesions has emerged. It has been variously termed 'phototherapy', 'photoradiation therapy', 'photodynamic therapy', and 'photochemotherapy'.

Although, currently, no photosensitizing drug is taken up or retained selectively only by malignant tissue, several potentially useful photosensitizers are available for which such a tumor-specific characteristic has been claimed. These include berberine sulfate, fluorescein, eosin, tetracycline, acridine organe, and several porphyrins [2–8]. Certainly the porphyrins have been the drugs most completely investigated, and they appear, at present, to be the most useful.

Hematoporphyrin is a product extracted by alcohol and sulfuric acid from hemoglobin, and was first discovered in the second half of the 19th century. Early investigators noted that hematoporphyrin tended to localize in malignant tissues, as could be noted from the fact that tumor cells would fluoresce a salmon-red color when exposed to ultraviolet light. However, observed tumor fluorescence was frequently inconsistent, resulting often in unreliable results. It was then ascertained that the hematoporphyrin product which was commercially available contained a mixture of porphyrins with varying localizing properties that in some cases exceeded those of pure hematoporphyrin. This prompted Lipson [4] to report on a method of preparing an acetic and sulfuric acid derivative of naturally occurring hematoporphyrin called 'hematoporphyrin derivative' (HpD) that showed a greater effect for malignant tissue than hematoporphyrin. It was subsequently found that HpD was not only a tumor localization agent, but also an active photosensitizing agent in that cytotoxicity would occur in cells that had taken up HpD if they were exposed to wavelengths of light corresponding to the absorption spectrum of HpD.

These early observations prompted us to explore the use of HpD, first as a tumor localization agent for transitional cell carcinoma of the bladder. Our subsequent fluorescence bladder mapping studies established that HpD does, indeed, localize preferentially in malignant and severely dysplastic transitional cells [9]. This fact, plus the knowledge that activation of intracellular HpD with light of appropriate wavelength results in cytotoxicity [10–19], prompted a trial of HpD photodynamic therapy in patients with focal and diffuse-resistant (Tis) of the urinary bladder.

Patients and Methods

Patient Selection

All patients had Tis that was resistant to conventional modalities of treatment. Most patients had undergone frequent fulgurations and also intravesical instillations of chemotherapeutic agents such as thiotepa, mitomycin C, and doxorubicin and had, nonetheless, experienced disease recurrence. Tis was confirmed by bladder biopsy, and all patients also had positive urinary cytologic examinations. All patients had been advised to undergo cystectomy and urinary diversion and had refused. The patients were treated under an experimental protocol previously approved by our institutional review board. There were 15 patients with focal Tis, and 15 patients with diffuse Tis (table I). Of the 15 patients with diffuse Tis, 2 also had focal T_2 disease (patients 9 and 10), and 2 (patients 1 and 8) had focal T_a lesions coexistent with their Tis. Patient 2 had diffuse Tis and also Tis within a large bladder diverticulum.

Light Irradiation Source and Optical Fibers

For focal treatment the optical guide used was a medical-grade quartz fiber, 5 m in length and having a core diameter of 400 µm. The exit beam divergence was approximately 20 degrees. The fiber was passed through the open channel of the endoscope, so that the distal end protruded from the tip of the instrument. During treatment the distal end of the fiber was positioned approximately 2–2.5 cm from the surface of the tumor. In this case the diameter of the beam was approximately 1 cm. In an attempt to increase the size of the intense spot, the distal tip of the fiber was formed into a microlens by heating in a flame. In this way the intense spot was spread over a diameter of 2 cm when the fiber was held 2–2.5 cm from the surface of the tumor.

The optical guide employed for whole-bladder therapy was a medical-grade quartz optical fiber with a core diameter of 400 µm. For light divergence, a spherical bulb made of clear polycarbonate was attached to the end of this fiber (fig. 1). With the fiber positioned approximately in the center of the bladder, the output of light in relation to the angle of impingement on the urothelium was that shown in figure 2. The overall coupling efficiency of the system was approximately 70% from laser to bulb, and the bulb efficiency was 96%; that is, 96% of the power in the fiber emerged from the bulb. The average output was 81% of the maximum recorded at any one point, and the rear octant was 50% of the average output (fig. 2). The rest of the field was within about 25% of the average value. These figures assumed that the bladder is a uniform sphere and did not take into account the reflectance of the bladder urothelium which is about 50% for red light. This reflectance should have resulted in a smoothing out of the light distribution.

The proximal end of the quartz fiber was attached to an optical positioning device which was coupled to the output of a continuous-wave dye laser. Adjustments were made so that the dye laser beam was focused directly into the optical fiber. Rhodamine B dye was circulated in the dye laser. The argon laser had a maximal power output of 20 W and was capable of producing an output of as much as 4 W at 630 nm from the dye laser.

Treatment Procedure

Focal. The hematoporyphyrin derivative employed was prepared in our laboratory by a modification of the technique of Lipson [4]. For initial treatment all patients received HpD intravenously at a dose of 2.5–5.0 mg/kg body weight approximately 3 h before light irradiation. Several patients were also given a second treatment 48 h after drug administration. Standard rigid cystoscopes equipped with the Storz laser fiber guide were used to deliver the light when possible. When lesions were located in the dome or at the bladder neck, a flexible fiberoptic bronchoscope or a flexible nephroscope-choledochoscope was used. Most procedures were done with the patient under general anesthesia. However, if the lesions were easily accessible and the patient requested it, treatment was performed with the patient under local anesthesia. All areas of Tis treated were $\leq$ 3 cm in diameter, although in a few cases the disease was multifocal. Even through the Tis were not $>$ 3 cm in diameter, the diameter of the light irradiation spot often was too small to cover the entire tumor when the probe was held in one position. However, all tumors seemed to be covered adequately by irradiating in two overlapping locations or by moving the probe slowly back and forth over the involved area. The light dose approximated 150 J/cm^2 for each treatment session and all treatment was performed at a wavelength of 630 nm. Patients were discharged from the hospital either the evening of the treatment day or the next morning.

Diffuse. All patients received 4–5 mg of HpD/kg body weight 3 h (initial 5 patients) to 48 h (subsequent patients) before exposure of the entire bladder to red light (630 nm) (table I).

Illumination times of approximately 60 min with power outputs of 1–1.5 W resulted in the delivery of 25–45 J/cm^2 to the entire urothe-

Table I. Whole-bladder HpD photodynamic therapy – patient history and treatment results

Patient No.	Age years	Sex	Pathologic findings	Previous therapy	Bladder capacity, cm^3	Response at 3 months	Follow-up time and status
1	70	M	multifocal Tis, grade 2; focal T_a	multiple fulgurations, thiotepa, Adriamycin, mitomycin C, focal HpD	150	partial (persistent T_a)	8 months repeat treatment: negative
2	75	M	multifocal Tis, grade 3	fulgurations, thiotepa	200	complete	6 months focal recurrence
3	72	M	multifocal Tis, grade 3	fulgurations, thiotepa, mitomycin C, Adriamycin	250	complete	9 months two low-grade papillary tumors fulgurated
4	76	M	multifocal Tis, grade 2	fulgurations, thiotepa, mitomycin C, focal HpD	250	complete	6 months negative
5	65	M	multifocal Tis, grade 2	fulguration, thiotepa, Adriamycin	150	complete	10 months negative
6	62	M	multifocal Tis, grade 2	fulgurations, thiotepa, mitomycin C, Adriamycin, focal HpD	180	complete	5 months negative
7	60	M	multifocal Tis, grade 3	fulgurations, partial cystectomy, thiotepa, mitomycin C	250	complete	7 months negative
8	60	M	multifocal Tis, grade 2; focal T_a	fulgurations, mitomycin C	180	partial (persistent T_a)	6 months negative
9	49	M	multifocal Tis, grade 3; focal T_2, grade 3	fulgurations, thiotepa, mitomycin C, Adriamycin	150	partial	8 months persistent T_2 disease
10	77	F	multifocal Tis, grade 3; focal T_2, grade 3	fulguration, thiotepa, mitomycin C, *cis*-platinum	200	partial	8 months cystectomy for recurrent disease
11	73	F	multifocal Tis, grade 3	fulguration, thiotepa	150	complete	6 months small, focal recurrent Tis fulgurated
12	72	M	multifocal Tis, grade 3	fulguration, thiotepa, mitomycin C, Adriamycin	200	complete	6 months negative
13	58	M	multifocal Tis, grade 3–4	fulguration, thiotepa	325		
14	67	F	multifocal Tis, grade 3	fulguration, mitomycin C	125		
15	58	M	multifocal Tis, grade 3	fulguration, thiotepa	250		

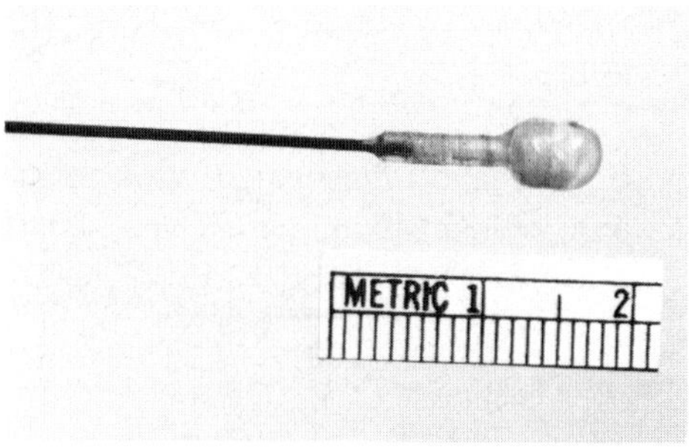

1

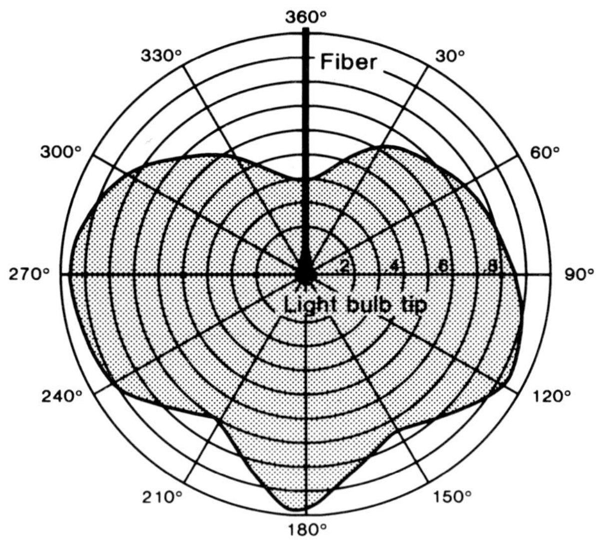

2

Fig. 1. Quartz fiber with a clear polycarbonate 'light bulb' tip. [From ref. 27, with permission.]

Fig. 2. Polar coordinate plot of relation of output to angle of light impingement on bladder urothelium. The bladder is assumed to be a perfect sphere. [From ref. 27, with permission.]

lium. All treatments were performed with general anesthesia and standard rigid cystoscopes equipped with a Storz laser fiber guide; saline was used as the irrigant. The fiber usually was placed as nearly as possible in the center of the bladder. The patient with both diffuse Tis and Tis in a bladder diverticulum (No. 2) was treated with the fiber in the center of the bladder for 60 min and in the center of the diverticulum for 30 min. On occasion, the fiber was located closer to the hemisphere of the bladder in which the disease was most prevalent in an attempt to increase the incident dose in the area of known tumor. This resulted in a diminished, but probably adequate, dose to the opposite, uninvolved hemisphere because of bladder reflectance.

Patient Follow-up and Interpretation of Results

All patients were informed of the need for close follow-up, including multiple cystoscopic and biopsy studies, to assess therapeutic response. After the initial treatment all patients were examined by cystoscopy at least once within the first 7 days after treatment. With experience we found that it takes at least 4 weeks for the initial edema and exudative reaction to subside before it is possible to obtain adequate revisualization, photographic documentation, and biopsy proof of the therapeutic result. Accordingly, the efficacy of HpD photodynamic therapy was determined by repeat cystoscopic examination and urinary cytologic examination and biopsy 3 months after treatment and every 3 months thereafter. (Biopsies were performed at these examinations if urine cytologic findings were positive or if a visual abnormality was present.)

Since the skin absorbs a quantity of hematoporphyrin derivative sufficient to produce marked photosensitivity, each patient was warned carefully and repeatedly to avoid exposure to bright light, especially direct and indirect sunlight, for up to 4 weeks.

Results

Focal Therapy

Cystoscopic examination in all patients 4–8 days after treatment revealed a pronounced exuberant local reaction characterized by edema, hemorrhage, and early necrosis. Biopsy at these times demonstrated a marked hemorrhagic and exudative reaction in the submucosal tissue and significant degenerative changes in the overlying urothelium. Thirty to sixty days after treatment, the mucosal surface was populated by essentially normal-appearing urothelial cells. All treated patients had biopsy and cytologic evidence of disappearance of the lesion in the treated area at the 3-month follow-up cystoscopic examination. Follow-up ranged from 6 to 32 months. Eight patients had one or more recurrent lesions, either in the treated area or in distant areas. In each case, the recurrence was successfully treated with HpD phototherapy. Two patients had five and six repeat treatments, respectively. One of the 15 patients underwent cystectomy and urinary diversion because of progression to T_1 disease after multiple recurrences.

The only adverse effect encountered was severe sunburn in 2 patients who did not heed warnings to remain out of direct or indirect sunlight.

Whole-Bladder Therapy

Of the 11 patients with Tis of the bladder alone, 8 patients have thus far returned for their 3-month follow-up evaluation, and all demonstrated complete disappearance of tumor (table I). Three of these eight patients have been noted to have focal recurrent disease (patient 2 at 6 months, patient 11 at 6 months, and patient 3 at 9 months after treatment). Two patients who had both Tis and T_a lesions were found to have disappearance of their Tis, but persistence of one (patient 1) or two (patient 8) T_a lesions at the 3-month follow-up examination. The 2 patients (Nos. 9 and 10) who had diffuse Tis and also focal invasive disease were noted to have persistence of invasive disease and disappearance of Tis. Patient 10 underwent cystectomy and urinary diversion. At the time of this report, patient 9, who had persistently refused cystectomy, is receiving systemic chemotherapy for metastatic disease.

Adverse effects of treatment were minimal. Cutaneous photosensitivity (sunburn), although a significant nuisance, was not severe in any of these patients. Specifically, the 2 patients who had undergone previous focal HpD photodynamic therapy did not experience any increased photosensitivity. Most patients noted bladder irritability characterized by frequency, urgency, and diminished bladder capacity shortly after therapy. This appeared to be more marked in patients treated 48 h after administration of HpD. Most patients had reduced bladder capacities before HpD photodynamic therapy (table I) due to their underlying disease and the types of previous therapy they had received. However, all patients reported that their subjective bladder capacity had returned to its pretreatment volume by the time of the first 3-month follow-up visit. Treatment results did not appear to be affected by pretreatment bladder volumes or by the timing of light delivery after administration of HpD (that is, whether at 3 or at 48 h).

Discussion

Several investigators have shown that HpD phototherapy has a significant antitumor effect in patients with Tis of the bladder [20–22]. In our early treatment attempts, a quartz fiber with a flat or slightly convex end was used, and the result was a spot of light only 2–2.5 cm in diameter. This small spot size greatly limited the area of tumor that could be treated at any one sitting. Our expanded series of 15 patients has confirmed the efficacy of focal HpD photodynamic therapy in patients with resistant Tis of the bladder, but the recurrence rates for patients with a field-change disease such as Tis of the bladder have remained significant. For this reason, our group and several others have investigated ways to deliver an ample amount of light to the entire bladder in hopes of reducing recurrence. Jocham et al. [23] introduced the possibility of the use of a lipid-diffusing medium, but no clinical trials in humans have been published. Hisazumi et al. [24] devised a laser light scattering optic coupled with a driving instrument that irradiates the entire bladder in sequential segmental strips. They used an argon ion, pumped dye laser as a light source in the treatment of 2 patients, delivering a dose of approximately 10 J/cm^2 to the entire bladder. Early results in these 2 patients appeared encouraging with urinary cytologic findings having returned to normal after treatment. This system, however, is cumbersome and costly.

We approached the problem of light delivery to the entire bladder by modifying the distal end of the delivery fiber. Our early attempts at forming a bulbous tip at the end of the fiber resulted in inadequate illumination at the bladder neck, but more recently we have used the previously described fiber with a 'light bulb' tip that delivers fairly uniform light to the entire bladder (fig. 1, 2). This fiber is simple and relatively inexpensive, and it allows significant light energy to be delivered. Although it has been suggested that as little as 10 J/cm^2 may be effective in the treatment of Tis, we prefer to deliver approximately 20 J/cm^2. However, formal dose-response relationships for HpD photodynamic therapy of Tis are not yet available.

The optimal dose of HpD and timing of light delivery for this disease are likewise unknown. Most authors have suggested the administration of 2.5–5.0 mg HpD/kg body weight. More recently, Dougherty et al. [25] separated HpD by gel exclusion chromatography and identified a new component of the mixture (dihematoporphyrin ether). The component was found to be responsible for the tumor-photosensitizing ability of HpD. It is possible that this new active component will be effective at lower doses and perhaps with less morbidity.

The timing of light delivery after HpD administration has varied in the few clinical studies reported dealing with the bladder. Most investigators treat between 48 and 72 h after administration of the drug. We occasionally treat as early as 3 h after giving the HpD and again at 48 or 72 h, if necessary. Early treatment was based on the appearance of bright fluorescence at 3 h in our bladder tumor localization studies and also in other tumor systems [9, 12, 26]. Recent studies in mice indicate that treatment before 3 h is ineffective and that the therapeutic effect reaches its maximum at 3 h and then levels off. Treatment at either 3 or 48 h in the present study was arbitrary and occasionally was based on patient convenience. None of the patients with diffuse Tis underwent fluorescence localization of the malignancy, because of its obviously diffuse nature and because of our conviction, based on previous studies, that HpD localizes in dysplastic and malignant transitional cells by 3 h after administration.

All the patients to whom we administered whole-bladder HpD photodynamic therapy had had multiple previous treatments of various types (table I) and, therefore, represented a highly select group of patients with resistant disease. We continue to believe that resistant Tis is the stage of disease best treated by HpD photodynamic therapy, and the present study confirms that it is possible to effectively treat not only diffuse disease, but also Tis in a bladder diverticulum. Traditionally, electrofulguration of lesions in a diverticulum has been somewhat worrisome because of the thinness of the wall and the fear of perforation or damage to adjunctive viscera. The light bulb fiber is easily inserted into a diverticulum, and appropriate light doses can be delivered without difficulty.

Comparison of treatment results with other therapeutic modalities is difficult, but it seems clear that our initial suspicion that patients with invasive disease are poor candidates for HpD photodynamic therapy, as it is currently delivered, is true (patients 9 and 10). Although we noted recurrence of tumor in 2 out of 8 patients with diffuse resistant Tis, we believe at this time that whole-bladder HpD photodynamic therapy holds promise in the treatment of this most difficult disease entity. Until more is known about the natural history and underlying causes of this problem, it may be naive to consider that any one treatment short of cystectomy will be curative. Perhaps consideration should be given to some form of adjuvant continuing therapy in combination with HpD photodynamic therapy for patients who refuse surgical therapy.

References

1 Blum, H.F.: Photodynamic action and diseases caused by light (Reinhold, New York 1941).

2 Auler, H.; Banzer, G.: Untersuchungen über die Rolle der Porphyrine bei geschwulstkranken Menschen und Tieren. Z. Krebsforsch. *53:* 65–68 (1942).

3 Figge, F.; Weiland, G.; Manganiello, L.: Cancer detection and therapy; affinity of neoplastic, embryonic, and traumatized tissues for porphyrins and metalloporphyrins. Proc. Soc. exp. Biol. Med. *68:* 640–641 (1948).

4 Lipson, R.L.: The photodynamic and fluorescent properties of a particular hematoporphyrin derivative and its use in tumor detection; thesis Mayo Graduate School of Medicine, Rochester (1959).

5 Mellors, R.; Glassman, A.; Papanicolaou, G.: A microfluorometric scanning method for the detection of cancer cells in smears of exfoliated cells. Cancer *5:* 458–468 (1952).

6 Moore, G.E.: Diagnosis and localization of brain tumors: a clinical and experimental study employing fluorescent and radioactive tracer methods (Thomas, Springfield 1953).

7 Policard, A.: Etude sur les aspects offerts par des tumeurs expérimentales examinées à la lumière de Wood. C.r. Séanc. Soc. Biol. *91:* 1423–1424 (1924).

8 Tomson, S.; Emmett, E.; Fox, S.: Photodestruction of mouse epithelial tumors after oral acridine orange and argon laser. Cancer Res. *34:* 3124–3127 (1974).

9 Benson, R., Jr.; Farrow, G.; Kinsey, J. ; Cortese, D.; Zincke, H.; Utz, D.: Detection and localization of in situ carcinoma of the bladder with hematoporphyrin derivative. Mayo Clin. Proc. *57:* 548–555 (1982).

10 Lipson, R.; Baldes, E.; Olsen, A.: The use of a derivative of hematoporphyrin in tumor detection. J,. natn. Cancer Inst. *26:* 1–8 (1961).

11 Lipson, R.; Baldes, E.: The photodynamic properties of a particular hematoporphyrin derivative. Archs Derm. *82:* 508–516 (1960).

12 Gregorie, H., Jr.; Horger, E.; Ward, J.; Green, J.; Richards, T.; Robertson, H., Jr.; Stevenson, T.: Hematoporphyrin derivative fluorescence in malignant neoplasma. Ann. Surg. *167:* 820–828 (1968).

13 Kelly, J.; Snell, M.: Hematoporphyrin derivative: a possible aid in the diagnosis and therapy of carcinoma of the bladder. J. Urol. *115:* 150–151 (1976).

14 Kinsey, J.; Cortese, D.; Moses, H.; Ryan, R.; Branum, E.: Photodynamic effect of hematoporphyrin derivative as a function of optical spectrum and incident energy density. Cancer Res. *41:* 5020–5026 (1981).

15 Gomer, C.; Dougherty, T.: Determination of [^{3}H]- and [^{14}C]-hematoporphyrin derivative distribution in malignant and normal tissue. Cancer Res. *39:* 146–151 (1979).

16 Diamond, I.; Granelli, S.; McDonagh, A.; Nielsen, S.; Wilson, C.; Jaenicke, R.: Photodynamic therapy of malignant tumors. Lancet *ii:* 1175–1177 (1972).

17 Dougherty, T.; Grindey, G.; Fiel, R.; Weishaupt, K.; Boyle, D.: Photoradiation therapy. II. Cure of animal tumors with hematoporphyrin and light. J. natn. Cancer Inst. *55:* 115–121 (1975).

18 Granelli, S.; Diamond, I.; McDonagh, A.; Wilson, C.; Nielsen, S.: Photochemotherapy of glioma cells by visible light and hematoporphyrin. Cancer Res. *35:* 2567–2570 (1975).

19 Dougherty, T.; Gomer, C.; Weishaupt, K.: Energetics and efficiency of photoinactivation of murine tumor cells containing hematoporphyrin. Cancer Res. *36:* 2330–2333 (1976).

20 Benson, R., Jr.; Kinsey, J.; Cortese, D.; Farrow, G.; Utz, D.: Treatment of transitional cell carcinoma of the bladder with hematoporphyrin derivative phototherapy. J. Urol. *130:* 1090–1095 (1983).

21 Tsuchiya, A.; Obara, N.; Miwa, M.; Ohi, T.; Kato, M.; Mayata, Y.: Hematoporphyrin derivative and laser photoradiation in the

diagnosis and treatment of bladder cancer. J. Urol. *130:* 79–82 (1983).
22 Hisazumi, H.; Misaki, T.; Miyoshi, N.: Photoradiation therapy of bladder tumors. J. Urol. *130:* 685–687 (1983).
23 Jocham, D.; Staehler, G.; Chaussy, C.; Schmiedt, E.; Unsöld, E.; Hammer, C.; Lohrs, U.; Brendel, W.; Gorisch, W.: Integrated dye laser therapy of bladder tumors after photosensitization with hematoporphyrin derivative (HpD). The use of a light-dispersion medium (Abstract). 78th Ann. Meet. Am. Urol. Ass., Las Vegas 1983, p. 155.
24 Hisazumi, H.; Miyoshi, N.; Naito, K.; Misaki, T.: Whole bladder wall photoradiation therapy for carcinoma in situ of the bladder; a preliminary report. J. Urol. *131:* 884–887 (1984).
25 Dougherty, T.; Boyle, D.; Weishaupt, K.; Henderson, B.; Potter, W.; Bellnier, D.; Wityk, K.: Photoradiation therapy – clinical and drug advances; in Kessel, Dougherty, Porphyrin photosensitization, pp. 3–15 (Plenum Press, New York 1983).
26 Lipson, R.; Baldes, E.; Olsen, A.: Hematoporphyrin derivative: a new aid for endoscopic detection of malignant disease. J. thorac. cardiovasc. Surg. *42:* 623–629 (1961).
27 Benson, R., Jr.: Treatment of diffuse transitional cell carcinoma in situ by whole bladder hematoporphyrin derivative photodynamic therapy. J. Urol. *134:* 675–678 (1985).

Ralph C. Benson, Jr., MD,
Department of Urology,
Mayo Clinic,
Rochester, MN 55905 (USA)

Eur. Urol. *12:* suppl. 1, pp. 54–57 (1986)

0302–2838/86/0127–0054$2.75/0

Experimental Investigation of Neodymium-YAG Laser Induced Shock Waves for Lithotripsy

F. Frank[a], *A. Hofstetter*[b], *E. Keiditsch*[c], *F. Wondrazek*[a]

[a] MBB-Medizintechnik GmbH, Applikationsforschung, München, BRD; [b] Urologische Klinik und Poliklinik der Medizinischen Universität zu Lübeck, BRD; [c] Institut für Pathologie, Klinikum München-Bogenhausen, München, BRD

Key Words. Lithotripsy · Neodymium-YAG laser · Optical breakdown · Optomechanical coupling · Shock waves

Abstract. Experiments on the endoscopic destruction of kidney stones by neodymium-YAG laser, either thermically or mechanically, are being carried out with various results. The thermal destruction is clinically not feasible, and the risk of damaging neighboring tissue is inevitable. The direct generation of shock waves with pulsed Q-switch systems seems to represent the only feasible endoscopic method subject to further development of suitable devices for clinical tests.

Introduction

It is generally recognized that extracorporeal shock wave lithotripsy has been revolutionary in simplifying the treatment of kidney stones and reducing the risks of therapy. The possibilities of the procedure are limited, however, in the case of deep-lying ureteral stones. Other methods, such as the use of ultrasound and Urat, have been unsatisfactory. In this connection the question arises as to the extent to which endoscopic destruction of kidney stones is possible with the neodymium-YAG (Nd:YAG) laser.

Thermal Stone Destruction

Both oxalate and uric acid stones can be incinerated, using the beam of continuous-wave lasers generally employed in urology [3] at power outputs of up to 100 W delivered through 0.6-mm quartz glass light guides [4]. Our 'in vitro' experiments showed that for irradiation under water the tip of the light guide must be placed directly on the stone in order to heat it to incandescence. Furthermore, as a result of fusing and formation of oxide, a pronounced change in the consistency of the surface of the stone occurs [2, 9].

In contrast to the views of Japanese researchers [5–7] we believe that 'in vivo' destruction of ureteral stones is impracticable. Because temperatures of up to 1,000 °C are generated, and irradiation times of up to 10 min are required, thermal and mechanical damage of the neighboring bladder and ureteral or renal pelvic tissue is inevitable.

Recently, experiments have been conducted using sapphire tips mounted on the end of the light guide, both to concentrate the laser radiation on the stone surface and to prevent destruction of the light guide tip. The results are not yet available [8].

Mechanical Stone Destruction

By using suitable resonator configurations, so-called 'Q-switch' arrangements, it is also possible to produce very short pulses of high intensity with a Nd:YAG laser. In this way power densities can be achieved at which an optical breakdown in gaseous, liquid, and solid media takes place. Extremely high local temperatures result, and shock waves are generated.

Other authors have succeeded in splintering off small fragments of the stone by focussing pulses of 1 J of energy and 20 ns duration [9] or pulses of 250 mJ and 1 ms duration [2] directly on the stone surface. However, in no case was complete fragmentation of the stones achieved.

The extent to which purely mechanical effects or thermomechanical tensile effects are involved here is unclear. Using pulses of 1 J of energy, no signs of thermal action, such as carbonization, were observed. It is certain, however, that with pulse times in the millisecond range thermal effects can no longer be ruled out. Attempts to induce resonance in the stone by means of suitable frequencies have not met with any success.

An endoscopic application with pulse energies of 250 mJ to 1 J and a pulse duration of several nanoseconds cannot be considered. The transmission of the laser light through conventional fibers having a diameter of 0.4–1 mm requires focussing. With such pulses the power densities developed destroy the fibers.

Fair [1], therefore, took up an idea of Yang [10] of converting light energy as efficiently as possible into mechanical energy. This method of optomechanical coupling is based on the production of shock waves by the absorption of the laser beam in an aluminum film. The aluminum film is situated on a glass cylinder which, in turn, is mounted in a brass cylinder. The explosion in the aluminum film resulting from the absorption of the laser pulse is transmitted to the stone by direct contact with the brass cylinder.

Using pulses of 14 mJ and 12 ns duration this optomechanical coupler is capable of disintegrating urinary stones; however, not only the stone, but also the aluminum film and the light guide are destroyed with each burst [2].

An estimate of the power densities occurring in the focussed coupling of Nd:YAG laser light in quartz glass light guides, as might be used in endoscopic urology, yields an irradiation limit of 1–2 GW/cm^2. In conjunction with the pulse times achieved with the electro-optical Q-switch system, namely 5–20 ns, this means that, depending on the diameter of the fiber, pulse energies of only 15–80 mJ can be used.

Our experiments were, therefore, designed to investigate whether efficient destruction of urinary stones in water is possible with laser-induced shock waves using pulse energies of 40–60 mJ. It is possible to generate such a shock wave with sufficient power density per pulse (approximately 6 GW/cm^2) directly in water.

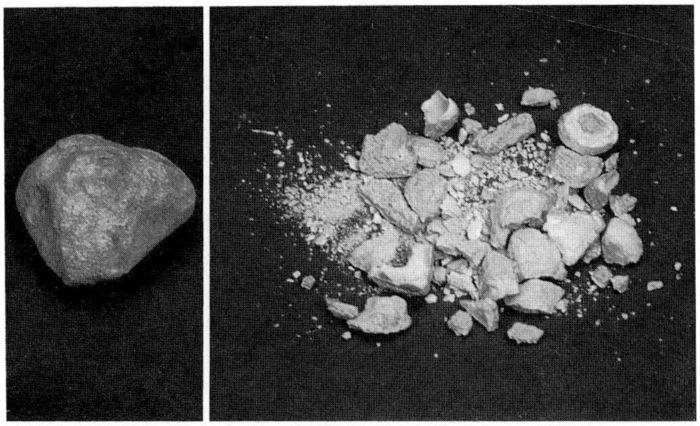

Fig. 1. Uric acid stone of approximately 1 cm^3 before (**a**) and stone debris after laser-induced shock wave treatment with 350 pulses (**b**). Pulse energy 45 mJ, pulse duration 6 ns.

Using a simple arrangement with a focussing system, a uric acid stone, about 1 cm^3 in volume, was gradually destroyed using about 350 pulses of 45 mJ and 6 ns duration. The stone debris ranged in size from dust-like particles to fragments of 2–3 mm. With the pulse frequency of 0.5 Hz inherent in the laser system used, a treatment period of about 15 min was required (fig. 1).

In a further step it proved possible with the help of a suitable coupling system to transmit pulses of 50 mJ through quartz glass fibers having a diameter of 1 mm and a length of approximately 5 m. The laser pulses were transmitted directly to the stone through the light guide and a distal coupling system. Depending on size and composition of the stone, 100–500 pulses of approximately 40 mJ were required to accomplish gradual destruction of the stones which were exposed under water. In order to include the elastic renal parenchyma in the process, the calculi were inserted into the incised kidneys of recently slaughtered pigs and destroyed under water (fig. 2).

Up to 40 pulses, likewise of 40 mJ, were delivered to the area of the cortex, the medulla, and the renal pelvis. The histologic examination in the near and far field revealed no evidence of mechanical structural damage to the renal parenchyma. To visualize fine structures, Gomori's silvering technique was employed (fig. 3). Neither the renal corpuscles nor the tubule system nor the urothelium showed grossly evident morphological changes.

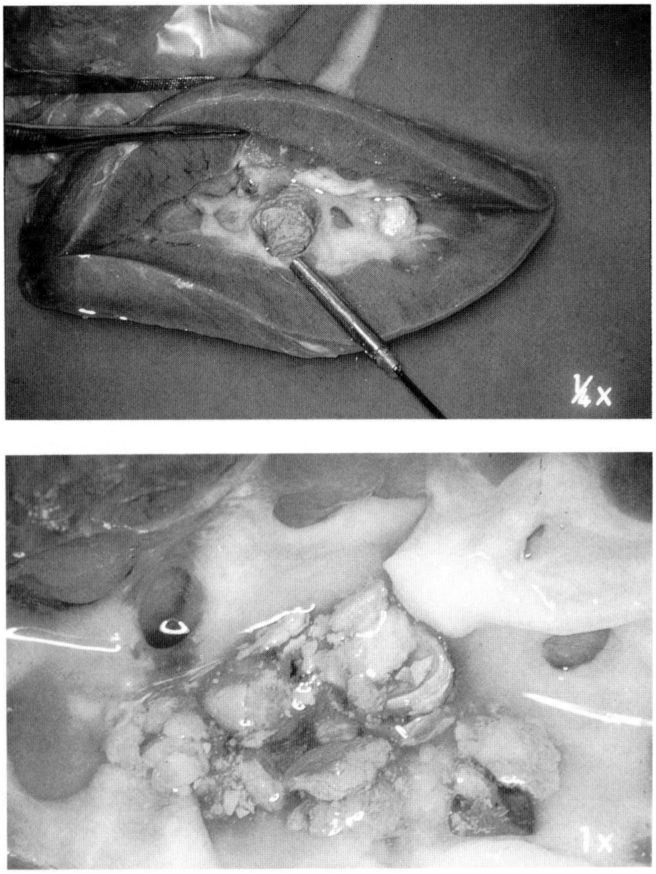

2a
2b

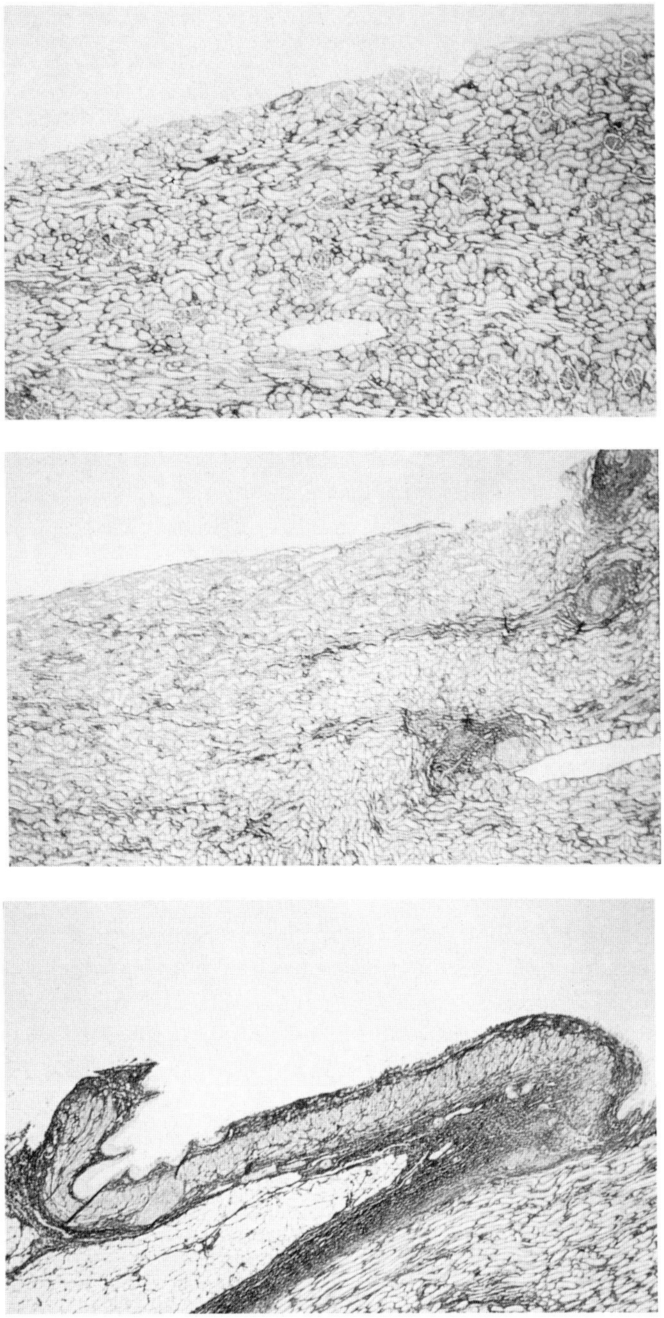

3a
3b
3c

Fig. 2. In vitro exposure of a kidney stone to laser-induced shock waves (**a**) and stone debris after 400 pulses (**b**). Pulse energy 40 mJ, pulse duration 6 ns.

Fig. 3. Area of the renal cortex (**a**), medulla (**b**), and pelvis (**c**) after exposure to 50 Nd:YAG laser pulses. Pulse energy 40 mJ, pulse duration 6 ns. Neither the renal corpuscles nor the tubule system shows any signs of damage.

Discussion

The thermal destruction of urinary stones with the Nd:YAG continuous-wave laser or with pulsed lasers in the millisecond range is not clinically feasible, since secondary damage to neighboring tissue is hardly avoidable. Work with optomechanical couplers in combination with laser pulses having energies of 10–20 mJ is not technically practicable.

Direct generation of shock waves with pulsed Nd:YAG Q-switch systems using energies of 40–60 mJ appears to represent the only feasible endoscopic method. Although it has been possible to transmit such pulses in the nanosecond range through conventional quartz glass fibers, suitable devices must be developed that permit visual control of the method before it can be clinically tested. The pulse frequency of the laser system employed must be increased to the extent that the required 200–500 pulses can be delivered within periods of 1–2 min. Histologically, in vivo animal experiments must establish beyond a doubt that no tissue damage is likely to occur.

Provided it proves appropriate for in vivo use, the technique could be of considerable clinical significance, since not only could it destroy ureteral stones, which are extremely difficult or impossible to treat by current therapeutic methods, but the principle could also be applied to other concrements, such as gallstones.

References

1 Fair, H.D.: In vitro destruction of urinary calculi by laser induced stress waves. Med. Instrum. J. *12:* 100–105 (1978).
2 Hofmann, R.; Schütz, W.: Zerstörung von Harnsteinen durch Laserstrahlung. Urologe A *23:* 181–184 (1984).
3 Hofstetter, A.G.; Böwering, R.; Keiditsch, E.; Frank, F.: Zerstörung von Uretertumoren mit dem Nd:YAG-Laser. Fortschr. Med. *101:* 625–627 (1983).
4 Pensel, J.; Frank, F.; Rothenberger, K.H.; Hofstetter, A.G.; Unsöld, E.: Destruction of urinary calculi by Nd:YAG laser irradiation. Proc. 4th Congr. Int. Soc. of Laser Surgery, Tokio 1981.
5 Tanahashi, Y.; Numata, I.; Kambe, K.; Harada, H.; Chiba, Y.; Toyoda, S.; Orikasa, S.: Transurethral disintegration of urinary calculi by use of laser beam. Proc. 4th Congr. Int. Soc. of Laser Surgery, Tokio 1981.
6 Tanahashi, Y.; Orikasa, I.; Numata, I.; Miyakawa, T.; Tahira, K.; Satoh, K.; Yamamoto, H.: The use of laser beam in Urology. Disintegration of extracted urinary calculi using optical waveguides. Jap. J. Urol. *71:* 28 (1980).
7 Tanahashi, Y.; Harada, K.; Numata, I.: J. Jap. Soc. Laser Med. *1:* 83 (1980).
8 Tanahashi, Y.; Chiba, Y.; Toyota, S.; Tasuchi, K.; Numata, J.; Orikasa, S.; Daikuzono, N.: Percutaneous laser lithotripsy of renal and uretric calculi using direct contact irradiation method. 2nd Nd:YAG Laser Conf., Munich 1985.
9 Watson, M.G.: Laser fragmentation of urinary calculi; in Smith, Laser in urologic surgery (Year Book Medical Publishers, Chicago 1985).
10 Yang, L.C.: Stress waves generated in thin metallic films by a Q-switched ruby laser. J. appl. Physics *45:* 2601–2608 (1974).

Dr. F. Frank,
MBB-Medizintechnik GmbH,
Postfach 80 11 68,
D–8000 München 80 (FRG)

Author Index

Subject Index